I0447987

Herbal Medicine

A Beginners Guide to Herbal Remedies
For
Health & Wellbeing

By

Dermot Farrell
www.healbodymindandspirit.com

1

Copyright © 2016 and beyond Dermot Farrell

All Rights Reserved.   No part of this publication may be reproduced in any form or by any means, including scanning, photocopying, or otherwise without prior written permission of the copyright holder.

Disclaimer and Terms of Use: The Author and Publisher has strived to be as accurate and complete as possible in the creation of this book, notwithstanding the fact that he does not warrant or represent at any time that the contents within are accurate due to the rapidly changing nature of the Internet. While all attempts have been made to verify information provided in this publication, the Author and Publisher assumes no responsibility for errors, omissions, or contrary interpretation of the subject matter herein. Any perceived slights of specific persons, peoples, or organizations are unintentional. In practical advice books, like anything else in life, there are no guarantees of income made. This book is not intended for use as a source of legal, business, accounting or financial advice. All readers are advised to seek services of competent professionals in legal, business, accounting, and finance field.

First Printing, 2016

MEDICAL DISCLAIMER

The information in this book is not intended to replace professional medical supervision. The information in this book is highly effective and it will definitely reduce the physical and mental health complaints of nearly every person, who earnestly uses the herbs and techniques outlined within. In some cases a cure may take place; however, there is no guarantee that physical ailments will be completely cured. Prior to reducing or stopping allopathic medications, do consult with a qualified physician.

Free Gifts

Bonus #1 – Grab Free Books!!!!!!!!

As a way of saying thank you for downloading this book I would like to give you two free books, which are available exclusively for my readers. The free book "Juicing for Health – 35 Juicing Recipes for Everyday Health Problems", is packed full of useful healthy juice recipes and Success Hacks - 31 Mind-Set Hacks to Increase Productivity and Career Success, is packed full of helpful mind hacks for developing a more dynamic and enjoyable lifestyle!

Please go to my blog page and sign up here:

www.healbodymindandspirit.com

You will receive the two free eBooks, plus weekly updates and even free eBooks!

Bonus#2 - Bonus Video Series

You can check out my YouTube channel, which has lots of health related videos

Please copy the following link into your browser, to access an introduction to herbal remedies video. If you then go to my channel and click playlists, you will find lots of videos on herbs for health:

http://y2u.be/rWpgVltW4dw

If you find it too awkward to type in this code, then you can also find my channel by typing in **www.healbodymindandspirit.com** into the YouTube search bar!

Table of Contents

Herbs have been widely used, throughout the generations, for a wide variety of health problems. Our ancestors may not have had our modern medical know how, but they still had health problems and they had to make some efforts to cure them. With the advent of modern pharmaceutical based medicine, there was a drop off in usage of natural herbal remedies. This drop off can be traced back to two factors; firstly the powerful effects of modern pharmaceuticals and secondly because of the corporate marketing, which backed this new pharmaceutical medical model.

Pharmaceuticals have certainly been effective, as the modern allopathic pharmaceutical model is presently dominating medicine with most general practitioners, hospitals and clinics, from all over the world distributing pharmaceutical drugs, in order to treat every imaginable condition. While we cannot argue that pharmaceutical drugs work, we must also realise that they also have their failings.

For a start modern drugs do not cure everything. Even if you are a strong proponent of the pharmaceutical model, it must be admitted that many people still suffer, even though there are so many drugs on the market today.

Furthermore, once modern drugs came on the scene their powerful effects made such strong waves that often older therapies and herbs were forgotten about. However, what everyone forgot during this medical revolution was that modern drugs come with a great many side effects and because modern drugs are so powerful, often the side effects are very strong which is contrary to the old style herbal remedies, which although weaker they were also less prone to side effects.

Another issue, with modern medicine is its fixation with treating symptoms rather than actually figuring out what is wrong with the patient. If two patients, for example, turn up to their doctor's office with acid reflux, more than likely the doctor will prescribe the exact same medication to them. However, if these patients go to a Traditional Chinese Medical practitioner, a Homeopath, a Naturopath or an Ayurveda practitioner, they will be asked many questions and the complimentary therapist will attempt to work out the aetiology (the cause) of the health imbalance. And more than likely the two patients will receive two different treatments, based upon their aetiology rather than on their symptoms!

Now modern medicine might well scoff, but why should they? Why is modern healthcare focused on treating symptoms, with little interest in finding the cause? Because modern medicine focuses so much on symptoms, it results in people who have several health problems receiving a barrage of medications, from doctors of different specialities. The cardiologist gives one drug, the diabetologist and gives another and then the stomach specialist gives yet another. Needless to say this mix of different drugs is rarely monitored by an overseeing doctor and as a consequence many side effects kick in, which in turn results in even more health imbalances.

This is not to say that modern medicine is bad, but rather that the "baby has been thrown out along with the bathwater". In an effort to modernise medicine, the old styled family physician, with a listening ear and a willingness to use a variety of therapies has gone. And in its stead, we have fancy multispecialty clinics and a plethora of screening tests. The patients are blood tested, put through ECT, Ultrasound, CAT scans, MRI's, Upper GI tests, lower GI tests and Colonoscopy. Yet for all this hi-tech medicine, in examining the patients, it is as if they were made out of pieces of LEGO, with each piece independent from each other one.

And yet in the background almost completely forgotten, by modern medicine, is a relic of a bygone age, an old system of medicine based upon rebalancing the health of the individual and using a variety of herbs and complimentary therapies, to bring about this balance. At last after nearly a century of pharmaceutical domination, individual health care workers from all over the world are starting to rediscover the value of these ancient treatment systems.

Why not use both old and new to treat our health problems!

Herbal remedies are not perfect. After all modern medicine is far more effective herbs in treating many conditions, but this does not mean that the herbs have no value. Just because we have added modern tech to healthcare, does not mean that we have to abandon the ancient treatments, why not use both old and new to treat our health problems!

Advantages and Disadvantages of Natural Herbal Remedies

Advantages:

•   Herbal remedies often produce a healing effect which is not possible with pharmaceuticals.

•   Some herbal remedies can replace pharmaceutical drugs, which are good for the body, as it reduces the possibilities of side effects, which often come with pharmaceutical drugs.

•   Even when pharmaceuticals cannot be completely replaced, often they can be reduced in dosage which in turn preserves the overall health balance of the body.

•   Pharmaceuticals are used to treat symptoms, but they do not fix the problem and often the underlying imbalance results in further health problems, over a long period of time.

•   Natural herbal remedies, on the other hand, often strengthen the body in a subtle way thus reducing further health complications.

Disadvantages:

18

• Herbs tend to be weaker, in effect, when compared with pharmaceutical medicine. This means that the pharmaceuticals can treat health conditions which the herbs cannot treat, but of course it also explains why allopathic medications produce so many side effects.

• Herbal remedies are slow to act. In this day and age we all want instant relief, but most herbs take time to work. In particular, for chronic health conditions, the herbs have to be taken on a daily basis for weeks before they become effective, so herbs require patience.

In summary herbs are very effective and one of the key things, with herbal remedies, is that they work with nature rather than against it, so they tend to protect the body from further health conditions, which cannot be said for pharmaceutical medicine.

However, there are some factors which must be taking into account, if you want to get the most out of natural herbal remedies:

Considerations:

1. Herbs are slow to work, so do not expect overnight results. In most chronic conditions, it will take several weeks of daily use before an improvement is noted. So it is really important that you don't just take some herbs, for a few days, and then scratch your head and conclude that they do not work. Rather pick a herb and give it a fair try out for a few weeks at least. Then add in other herbs in a systematic approach.

2. Remember that the great advantage, with herbs, is that not only are they cheap and effective but also they have health sparring properties, whereas allopathic drugs definitely result in toxicity and side effects over time, and often they result in other negative health conditions, because they do not address the health imbalance rather they just patch up the symptoms. Allopathic medicine is

basically like a band aid. Yes a band aid has its place but we have to treat the health imbalance, if we want to really look after our wellbeing. Herbs though slow to work are worth a little bit of patience.

3.   Herbal remedies tend to be weaker. Because of this they have less toxicity and side effects which is great, but on another level it also means that not only are they slower to work but usually several herbs have to be combined in order to be truly effective.

4.   After outlining the wonderful natural approach to treating your health conditions, a little reality checking is also necessary. Herbs contain chemical compounds, which are often very effective, but also they can be toxic and even if they are not toxic, they can have interactions with drugs, which are hazardous to our health. With this in mind, in this book we have included contraindications for each herb, so always take a look at the contraindications.

5.   Another thing which must also be borne in mind is possible allergic reactions, so always start off with a small dose and build up over a few days or so, in order to make sure that the herb works well for you. Don't just say "aw they're just herbs", no they're not just herbs, rather they are powerful medical compounds, so while very safe, in general, be careful be safe.

A Final Note on Herbal Dosing – Processed Herbs Versus Raw Herbs

Herb dosing is an important thing to keep in mind when taking herbs.

Firstly, raw herbs are a lot more powerful than herbs out of a bottle. There are lots of reasons why processed herbs will be less powerful, but it is an important consideration, as when it is a choice between processed versus raw always go with raw, but do take care as they are powerful!

Secondly, the majority of herbs mentioned in this book come straight out of your kitchen, which is great. Your kitchen herbs can save your life, literally! But also they are obviously very safe to take. For example, have you ever heard of someone overdosing on garlic? Not likely! So most herbs are very safe to take. But some herbs are very potent and great care has to be taken.

Always read the contraindications section of each herb listed and take care, and in particular some herbs mentioned in this book are really powerful and have to be respected, in the same way which you would respect allopathic medicine.

Never think that "it's only a herb" and it won't be effective or it won't have any potential risks. Herbs really are effective and also have to be treated with respect!

Herbal Remedies Have Been Clinically Tested and Proven Effective

For those of you who are sceptical of herbs and their effectiveness, footnotes are included throughout this book, which will refer the reader back to the footnote section, where a large list of clinical trials, have been referenced. A great number of scientific clinical trials have been carried out on so many herbs and in many cases they have been scientifically proven to work!

Also, for easy access, two appendixes have been added. Appendix one is a quick guide to the various herbal teas, infusions, tinctures and so on, which have already been mentioned in each chapter. If you want to skip over chapters and go straight to the herbal remedies, then just take a quick look through appendix one.

In appendix two, the various herbs mentioned in this book are listed, along with an extensive list of healing properties. For the sake of brevity, in this book certain prominent herbs have been selected and an emphasize has been placed upon their healing significance, in one or more health conditions. However, each of these herbs can potentially treat far more health conditions. So if you have a health condition and just want a quick reference guide to the herbs which can help this condition, then take a look through appendix two.

So hopefully by now, you are eager to see the herbal remedies and to give them a try. Do please remember the points noted above. Start slowly and stick with it for a few weeks, so as to give the herbs a chance to work. Finally try to use more than one herb, so as to provide a good overall effect, as herbs tend to work in a slow and gentle manner.

Another consideration, to think about, is what else can be done to help your health. Maybe a trip to a complimentary therapist could be a good idea or at least consider doing some yoga, tai chi or chi gong, in order to rebalance your health. In most cases, when we have a health problem it did not start over night, rather ill health is nearly always built upon a foundation of health imbalances. So think about taking a holistic approach.

Finally do take responsibility for your health. Chances are that if you are reading this book, probably you have some health problem or problems, which modern health care is not addressing properly. So if you just drop into your local multispecialty clinic, chances are that you're just another number. The prescribing physician is likely stressed out and over worked and will usually try to fix you within a 15 minute visit!

If you want to get of off this particular fairground ride, then take responsibility for your health. Now taking responsibility can be a challenge, because it means reading health books, trying out herbal remedies, visiting complimentary therapists and yes making lifestyle changes, such as taking out a gym membership and tidying up your diet. But this is what it takes. There are only two options:

A)   Be a patient and test your patience while the modern healthcare system processes you.

B)   Take responsibility, which means going on a journey of self-discovery. Trying different things out and learning by trial and error.

This book isn't simply another book with a list of cool herbs; rather the intention of this book is to challenge you, the reader, to take a novel approach to treating your own health. Also, we are not advocating dumping the allopathic pharmaceutical health system; rather it's about using common sense and trying out allopathic and complimentary approaches, to treating your health.

For too long a time allopathic healthcare practitioners have been at odds with complimentary therapists and vice versa, and all of this is silly. Here's a line out of the modern version of the Hippocratic Oath, the oath which is taking by many doctors during graduation today:

"I will remember that there is art to medicine as well as science, and that warmth, sympathy, and understanding may outweigh the surgeon's knife or the chemist's drug."

It is high time to go beyond the fighting and rather move forward, in an integrative way towards helping the patients to regain their health. And readers, may you also be encouraged to challenge yourself to investigate herbal remedies and give them a fair trial, you may well be pleasantly surprised by the results!

Chapter Two - Anxiety

Kava Kava

Kava kava is a medicinal plant (Piper methysticum) which comes from the south pacific Islands, where it has been used for centuries as a cure for anxiety, depression, insomnia and other mental health issues.

The active ingredients are Kavalactones, which have been well researched and have been proven effective at treating anxiety and other General Anxiety Disorders (GAD). According to research carried out in Australia 1, the kava kava plant brings about a significant reduction in anxiety symptoms in their test group. This study lasted eight weeks and involved 160 participants, 37% of the kava kava group demonstrated a noticeable response. The test group was sub divided into two groups, one group which were giving the actual kava kava and a second group which were given a placebo. By the end of the study, the participants who took the real kava kava, demonstrated a significant reduction in anxiety. Of particular interest, 26% of the kava kava group were still in remission of their anxiety symptoms!

Thirty seven percent of participants went in to remission from anxiety and depressive symptoms

Furthermore, during this study the participants were given anywhere from 120mg to 240mg of kava kava and none of the participants suffered issues regarding the quantity of the kava which they were taken. From this it can be concluded that kava kava is well tolerated, by the body, over a period of time.

25

Interestingly, kava kava not only produces a significant decrease in anxiety related issues, but it is largely free of side effects, unlike its medicative equivalents.

Is Kava kava safe?

Kava kava was banned from many countries in Europe back in 2002. However, in early 2014, this ban was lifted. The ban was enforced because of a spate of patients who suffered from liver damage, after taking kava kava. However, in 2014 the German high court overturned the ban, following an investigation of evidence which demonstrated only a tenuous link between kava kava and liver hepatoxity.

Kava kava is more than likely safe to use; after all it has been widely used by the south pacific islanders for hundreds of years, without any negative consequences. However, it must always be borne in mind that herbs, while naturally occurring do possess chemicals which could cause some negative side effects or even toxicity. One must always be careful when imbibing anything into one's body, even if it be a herb. But it must also be noted that western pharmaceuticals have a pretty poor record, when it comes to side effects. And a great many people who take anti-anxietic and anti-depressive drugs, will testify to the considerable negative side effects, which often come along with the drug.

How to take Kava kava:

Traditionally it is either chewed, or ground and squeezed and then added to beverages. Today kava kava, usually comes either as a pill or a powder. You can of course eat the kava kava root raw, but this will probably not be palatable to most people.

Pills are easy to take but tend to be less effective, because of fillers required in the pill making process.

The most effective way to take kava kava is in powder form. Take a beverage and mix two table spoons of kava kava. Using a mixer, mix thoroughly, then filter (to get rid of any sediment), and drink.

A tablespoon is approximately 15grams in size, so one helping (2 tablespoons) is around 30grams of kava kava. Kava kava can be taken several times a day, but obviously don't go overboard and start taking hundreds of grams a day. Start off with one serving a day and after a few days increase the amount if it feels ok, if any negative symptoms arise back of or even stop. As always, one man's poison is another man's meat, so start small and see how it goes. Also, reduction in symptoms will not be instantaneous, give it a couple of weeks and then assess to see whether symptom relieve has come about or not.

In particular, kava kava is very helpful at curing insomnia, so starting out, try it out an hour before bedtime and there is a good chance of an improved night's sleep. Also, once anxiety levels start to reduce and emotions improve, back of the amount of kava kava been imbibed. Think of it this way, initially start with a small amount and run it for a few days so as to assess the body's tolerance levels. If the tolerance levels are good, then increase the frequency to two servings per day (this can further be increased to three if need be). As mental tensions are relieved, observe how your state is improving.

After a while the rate of improvement will level off, at this stage the frequency of kava kava servings can be reduced. The idea behind this is one of following a testing phase, a loading phase and then a maintenance phase. Even with herbs, try and use as little as is necessary in order to get the job done!

Kava Kava Tea

1.   Take 3tbsp's of kava kava in with 3 cups of water.

2.   Heat for 5 minutes.

3.   Strain and pour.

Also, Kava Kava can be mixed with sprite or 7up or even coconut milk!

Kava Kava Contraindications:

•   Aprazolam (Xanax) causes drowsiness. When combined with kava kava this could bring about excessive drowsiness levels.

•   •   Levodopa increases dopamine levels in the brain, while kava brings dopamine levels down. Consequently, kava kava might reduce the effectiveness of levodopa in some cases.

St John's Wort

St John's Wort (Hypericum perforatum) is a perennial plant which has been used to treat nerve disorders, over the last two thousand years. St John's Wort, is found in Europe, Asia and the USA. The petals and leaves contain a variety of substances including hyperforin and hypercin.

Hyperforin is a substance which is good for spasm reduction in the gastro intestinal tract2.

Also, it is the main chemical substance found in St John's wort and has been found to have a strong anti - depressive action. In a 1998 study of 147 subjects (Laakman et al., 1998), subjects who were giving hyperforin demonstrated a significant reduction in depressive symptoms, in comparison to the placebo group. 3

Hypercin, displays a wide range of healing benefits which includes wound healing and anti-inflammatory treatment4, antimicrobial effects5, sinusitis treatment6, and seasonal adjustment disorder (SAD)7.

It can be noted that St. John's Wort, is not simply an anti-depressive, rather it has a curative effect on a wide range of health conditions. St John's Wort is also one of the most researched herbs and the results across more than thirty studies have confirmed its beneficial effects on mild depressive symptoms.

How exactly St John's Wort works, is still something of a mystery, although some researchers suggest that it has a beneficial effect on serotonin levels in the brain, serotonin been the feel good hormone which is commonly released either after exercise or injury. This could also explain why St John's Wort is so effective at treating SAD, as one of the key causes of Seasonal Adjustment Disorder is the reduction in exposure to sunlight in the winter months, which in turn reduces serotonin levels.

How to take St John's Wort:

St John's Wort, can be made into a tea, via its dried leaves or it can be taken in liquid or capsule form and the usual dosage is 300mg, three times a day. As always, with herbs start of on a low amount, like one serving per day, for a few days, in order to assess whether the body has any negative reactions to the herb, then increase to three times daily and once relief has come, back off slightly. As always take the minimum dosage required for a beneficial effect.

Contraindications:

•   It is safe to take St John's Wort, as it has been used for hundreds of years, so it obviously works. However it tends to interact with other drugs and make them less effective. So make a point of taking St John's Wort a couple of hours before or after allopathic medications.

•   Do not take St John's Wort with Selective serotonin reuptake inhibitors (SSRIs). . These are anti-depressant which work by boosting serotonin levels, and when combined with St Johns Wort, can result in to much serotonin, which result in serotonin syndrome, which could make you very sick or even prove to be fatal!..On a good note though it also means that St Johns Wort may help to relieve depression, as it boosts serotonin!

•   Avoid if using anti-convultants, oral contraceptives, , theophylline, warfarin, digoxin, , triptans or HIV protease inhibitors.

•   Do not take when pregnant or when breastfeeding.

•   Avoid over exposure to the sun if fair skinned.

Valerian

Valerian is found both in North America and Europe. Valerian has been used for centuries for the

treatment of anxiety, insomnia as well as a way of relaxing muscle tension.

The active ingredient in valerian is valerenic acid. Valerenic acid has been noted for having a variety of benefits which include antioxidant properties, liver protection properties, treatment of insomnia and also for the treatment of anxiety. In two studies, one on GABA8 and one on 5-HT5A receptor activity9, note a noticeable improvement in the activity of potentiating and inhibiting the GABA receptors as well as stimulating the 5-HT5A receptor. Both of these physiological activities relate back to anxiety and its possible reduction via valerenic acid.

Sleep benefits have also been noted, in the way that valerenic acid has a positive effect on treating insomnia. In a study of 16 participants a noticeable improvement in sleep patterns emerged. 10

Also, note that often people who suffer from anxiety symptoms and symptoms of depression, have difficulty sleeping. Enhancing sleep will often aid mood enhancement and possible this is one of the reasons why valerian is so effective at treating anxiety and depression.

How to use Valerian:

Valerian usually comes in tablet form, or it can come as a dry herb. Most pills contain 400mg of valerian. For insomnia a dosage anywhere between 400mg to 900mg per day, one hour before bedtime. In the case of anxiety a higher dosage can be taken, a dosage of 400mg three times a day can be taken, without any negative side effects. If using the valerian root, then use one to two grams of the root, mixed with tea, up to three times a day. In treatment of children use a dosage based upon their bodyweight. Also, valerian is fairly slow to act, so give it a couple of weeks before expecting a noticeable result.

Valerian tends to be well tolerated, but like all herbs start low, and if all is well then build up and then back of back to a maintenance dose. Use enough to produce a good result, more is not always better.

Contraindications:

- Do not take while on sleeping medication.

- Do not take if pregnant or breastfeeding.

- Do not use before driving or using heavy machinery.

Passionflower

Passionflower is native to South America, but it is also found widely throughout Europe. Like the other herbs mentioned above, it has been widely used, over the years, as a means of sedation and relaxation. It contains glycosides, alkaloids as well as steroids. In particular it is the alkaloids which have a beneficial effect on mood enhancement.

In a 2002 study of 36 patients, who suffered from General Anxiety Disorder (GAD), the group was split into a placebo group, an oxazepam group (anti-anxietic) as well as a passionflower group. By the end of the study, it was concluded that oxazepam acted more rapidly than the passionflower, but it also came with far more side effects. However, apart from a quicker onset of relief, from anxiety, the end result was the same level of relief from anxiety using either oxazepam or passionflower!

How to Take Passionflower:

Passionflower comes in a liquid form as a tincture which can be taken at 1.4ml three times a day, or it can be taken as a dry root, in which case 0.5grams to 1gram can be taken three times a day, mixed in a tea. In the case of tea place a dry root into the water and boil for ten minutes before straining and then drinking.

Passionflower Tea

1. Grind 2 grams of passionflower (per cup) into a fine powder.

2. Add the ground leaves into a cup of water and bring to the boil.

3. Leave to simmer for 20 minutes.

4. Strain and drink.

Passionflower Tincture

1. To make a tincture, we have to mix the plant material with a liquid which will suck out the chemical compounds from the herb, this liquid is called the menstruum. The ratio necessary with is 2:1. The menstruum is usually alcohol, but apple cider vinegar can be used instead. The menstruum also also helps to preserve the tincture, so the tincture can be used over a long period of time. Brandy, vodka, and grain alcohol are used as the alcohol base, do not use beer! It's necessary for the menstruum to be high in alcohol, so as to preserve the tincture.

2.   To make the menstruum, mix in alcohol/apple cider vinegar to a ratio of 3:1 with water and the menstruum with the passionflower with a ratio of 2:1.

3.   Take 3 ounces (90grams) of alcohol/vinegar to a ratio of about 1 ounce (30 grams) of water. Then place the mix into a blender and blend. The flower now has to be chopped and ground. Then add in 2 ounces (60grams) of passionflower with 4 ounces (120 grams) of menstruum.

4.   Then pour into a glass container (do not use plastic), and leave it in a dark cool place.

5.   Shake every day for the next 14 days.

6.   Strain through several layers of cheesecloth and squeeze out the essence.

7.   Leave the mix which remains to settle for 12 to 16 hours, then pour out the clear liquid from the top of the jar, which is called the decant.

8.   The decant can now be Stored in a dark glass container in a dark place which should also be cold.

When you want to take it just take out a tincture dropper and use one to two drops anywhere, three to five times daily.

This tincture will last a long time because of the preserving qualities of alcohol/vinegar.

Contraindications:

Do not take if pregnant or breastfeeding.

Chamomile (matricaria recutita (German chamomile) and chamaemelum nobile (Roman chamomile)) is famous as a relaxing tea, but what many people do not know is that chamomile is also an effective anti-anxiety drug. A hundred years ago, before the advent of anti-depressants and anti-anxiety drugs, doctors used to recommend chamomile tea as a good way to treat depression and anxiety related symptoms. Chamomile is widely found through Europe and has been used since the time of the Pharaohs, for the treatment of anxiety and depression.

Chamomile produces an oil which contains 28 different types of terpenoids, including bisabolol, chamazulene and 36 flavonoids, which include luteolin as well as quercetin, which are natural anti-inflammatory agents and natural antioxidants.

In action chamomile has been found to have a positive effect on a wide variety of health conditions including insomnia, inflammation, skin conditions and even stomach problems. Regarding relief from symptoms of anxiety, in a 1995 study they noted that "the aqueous extract of this plant led to the detection of several fractions with significant affinity for the central benzodiazepine receptor and to the isolation and identification of 5,7,4'-trihydroxyflavone (apigenin) in one of them.".…….. and that The results reported in this paper demonstrate that apigenin is a ligand for the central benzodiazepine receptors exerting anxiolytic and slight sedative effects but not being anticonvulsant or myorelaxant."[12] In layman's language, chamomile binds to the benzodiazepine receptor in the same manner that an antidepressant will, but chamomile is of course a natural product with very few side effects!

How to take Chamomile:

Chamomile can either be drunk as a tea via a manufactured tea bag or it can be handmade. Needless to say, the handmade version will usually be more efficacious. When using a teabag, try out a few producers and see the effects, many times a herbal tea will have nice packaging but the quality will be low. If it is a good quality product, noticeable relief in stress will be found within minutes of drinking the tea.

In the case of a homemade tea, it can be made by taking one heaped teaspoon of dried flowers in a pot of boiled water and steeped for ten minutes. Strain it and drink it and add lemon or honey for taste.

Chamomile Tea

1.   Boil water.

2.   Add one teaspoon of dried chamomile leaves.

3.   Simmer for twenty minutes.

4.   Strain and serve.

Contraindications:

•   Watch for excessive drinking of chamomile tea during pregnancy, otherwise it is generally safe to take.

Butterbur

Butterbur (petasites hybridus) has been used by the Native Indians and Europeans to treat headaches and inflammation and allergies, for hundreds of years. In a study comparing butterbur with cetirizine, it was found that there was significant difference between the two regarding their effectiveness. Also, in favour of butterbur it managed to relieve symptoms, without creating the drowsiness which comes when using citrizine. 1

Leukotriene's are inflammatory mediators which set off allergic rhinitis. Presently drugs known as leukotriene modifiers are used to prevent allergic rhinitis and asthma symptoms from occurring. In another study carried out in 2001, it was noted that petasites have an inhibiting effect on the synthesis of leukotriene. 2 Since butterbur contains a large quantity of patasines, this explains why butterbur is so effective at testing allergies.

It can further be noted that butterbur has also been found as an effective treatment for migraines3 and asthma. 4

How to take Butterbur:

Butterbur is usually taken in capsule form, so the petasines have to be extracted, as raw butterbur contains pyrrolizidine alkaloids (PAs) which can cause liver damage, so it is safer to stick with the capsules.

Usually three to four 50mg capsules per day will produce a good result. Butterbur is usually well tolerated, but it must be remembered that allergic medications only need to be taken when the allergy is present. So it is best practice to avoid taking butterbur, if no symptoms are present and then taken as needed when symptoms arise, as this will reduce the chances of developing any side effects.

Contraindications:

• Butterbur can be toxic to people who have liver disease, so avoid in this case.

• Butterbur can also result in an allergic reaction in people who are sensitive to ragweed, marigolds, daisies and chrysanthemums.

• When giving to children reduce the dosage according to body weight and monitor for any negative side effects.

Quercetin

Quercetin is a flavonoid, flavonoids are plant pigments which give glowers, fruits and vegetables their particular colors.Flavonoids are antioxidants, antioxidants kill off free radicals which in turn is good for health.

However, unlike other flavonoids, Quercetin has some unusual properties. Quercetin stops immune cells from releasing histamines, which in turn stops allergic reactions in their tracts. The action takes place by inhibiting the release of lysosomal beta-glucuronidase, which is brought about by neutrophils. According to a 1984 study (Bosse et al.), Quercetin was one of only two flavonoids which

38

acted this way, the other been chalcone. A second observation was also made, noting that Quercetin suppressed the generation of superoxide anion by neutrophils.5 In layman's language an allergic reaction takes place because the body over reacts to a potential treat, to such a degree that the body's reaction becomes symptomatic. In the case of quercetin, it acts in two different ways in order to suppress this over active response.

How to take Quercetin:

Quercetin comes in pill form, usually around 500mg per pill, and it can be taken from one to three times daily. In the case of allergies, it is usually a good idea to space out the servings throughout the day, so as to prolong the beneficial effects for as long as possible. As always take as little as is necessary, in order to get the job done. Quercetin is well tolerated by most people, however, in some case large doses produce some side effects and even toxicity in the kidneys.

It' also worth noting that quercetin can be imbibed organically by eating vegetables which are high in quercetin, such as:

- Broccoli

- Capers

- Kale

- Raw asparagus

- Raw red onions

Also the following herbs, are all high in quercetin:

- St. John's Wort

- American Elder

- Ginkgo Balboa

But it must also be noted that unless vast amounts of these vegetables and herbs are ingested, some supplementation may still be needed, as while 500mg a day can easily be ingested via food, however, a higher dosage such as 1000mg might not be so easy to take.

Contraindications:

- Avoid if breastfeeding or pregnant.

- High dosages can be kidney toxic, so should be avoided by kidney patients.

- Sometimes causes headaches or tingling in the arms and legs, if these symptoms are noted reduce the dosage or stop taking it as necessary.

Stinging nettle

Stinging nettle (Urtica dioica and Urtica urens) grows in Europe and North America and has been used as an herbal remedy for thousands of years. Stinging nettle is famous for its nettles and their painful sting, however, it also has a really good effect on allergic reactions by inhibiting histamine activity.6

In a 1990 study of 98 subjects, which was run through the hay fever season (May until early July), the group was split into placebo and nettle group. In the nettle group, 32% reported a dramatic improvement in symptoms and 84% reported a moderate improvement in symptoms. 7

How to take Stinging Nettle:

Stinging nettle comes in a variety of ways, which includes capsules, herbs and tea. Capsules usually come in 500mg and can be taken up to several times a day. Stinging nettle can also come as a tea, in a teabag, but this is very weak. In herbal from a couple of teaspoons of the herbal powder can be mixed either with hot water or a beverage.

A good option, if you have time is stinging nettle in raw, whereby you make your own tea, via actual dried nettles.

Stinging Nettle Tea

1.   Add 1ounze (28grams) of stinging nettle powder.

2.   Boil water

3.   Add stinging nettles to the water and leave to simmer for 20 minutes.

4.   Strain and serve.

Stinging Nettle Infusion

1.   Half fill a pint sized jar with dried nettles.

2.   Add boiling water. Secure the lid, using some wax paper so as to seal in the vapour.

3.   Let the jar sit for at least 4 hours.

4.   Filter and place the infusions in a glass jar and keep in the refrigerator.

The stinging nettles infusion can be heated up and drank just like a tea, the only difference been that the infusion is much stronger than the herbal tea. Experiment with each and see how it feels for you.

Stinging nettle tea and infusions will keep for 3 to 4 days.

Another option is to make a tincture, with a tincture alcohol is added so to preserve the herb for longer. Also, the final product, the tincture requires ten in drops.

To make a tincture, start off by finely cutting the dried nettle leaves add fill a large glass jar to the top with nettles, and then pour vodka or gin or rum over the nettles until the jar is filled. Please note that if you do not want to use alcohol as a base then apple cider vinegar can be used instead.

Next place wax paper over the lid, to make a better seal and then close the lid. Then place the jar in a dark place for a minimum of one month, in order to cure.

If possible leave it for a longer time period as the longer time period will make it stronger. Also, shake the bottle twice each day, so as to mix the ingredients. When ready to use, open the bottle and strain the solution form the leaves, and place the remnant into a bottle. One teaspoonful is enough for one serving.

Contraindications:

•   Stinging nettles should not be used by pregnant ladies or ladies who are breastfeeding.

•   Stinging nettles increase urine flow so beer in mind in the case of kidney patients.

•   Singing nettles can lower blood sugar, so a point to bear in mind for diabetics. Also, a good reason for taking it!

•   Stinging nettles can lower blood pressure, so in some cases this can result in lo BP. Also this means that it's a good herb for high blood pressure patients!

Thyme for Cold Relief

Thyme (thymus vulgaris) is an evergreen herb which grows in countries, all over the world, and is probably one of the most popular herbs because of its use as a culinary herb. However, as well as adding taste to food, thyme is also of great medicinal use. The leaves possess antibacterial, antimicrobial, anti-viral and astringent properties. Thyme is also really good at treating stomach problems and bronchial symptoms.

The leaves of the thyme plant possess a huge amount of healing compounds, which includes apigenin, bomeal, carvacrol, caffeic acid, flavonoids, labiatic acid, luteolin, oleanolic acid, saponins and ursolic acid.

Thyme is quite famous as a home remedy for a wide range of ailments, including high blood pressure treatment, immune system boosting, mouth cleansing and for the treatment of bronchial infections. Regarding bronchial relief, research backs up its effectiveness as a bronchial treatment. In a study of 361 patients, using an infusion of thyme and ivy, versus a placebo group, they found that the coughing fits in bronchial patients, relative to baseline, by day seven to nine, stopped in the case of 68.7% of thyme-ivy infusion patients versus only 47.6% of the patients, in the case of the placebo group. 1

How to take Thyme:

Thyme is usual taken as a tea. Add two teaspoons thyme to boiling water, steep for ten minutes, strain and drink. Take up to four servings per day, until symptoms clear.

Another option is a tincture of twenty to fourth drops (one to two ml) up to three times daily.

Thyme Tea

1.   Add 2 tbsps. of fresh thyme to 1 cup if boiling water.

2.   Steam for 10 minutes.

3.   Filter and serve.

Exotic Version of Thyme Tea

1.   Add 2 tbsps. of fresh thyme to 1 cup if boiling water.

2.   Steam for 10 minutes.

3.   Add 1 tbsp. of honey, 1 tsp. of turmeric, 1 tops of cayenne paper and 1 tsp. of grated ginger.

4.   Add 1 tbsp. of lemon juice.

5.   Filter and serve.

Thyme Tincture

1.   To make a tincture, we have to mix the plant material with a liquid which will suck out the chemical compounds from the herb, this liquid is called the menstruum. The ratio necessary with is 2:1. The menstruum is usually alcohol, but apple cider vinegar can be used instead. The menstruum also also helps to preserve the tincture, so the tincture can be used over a long period of time. Brandy, vodka, and grain alcohol are used as the alcohol base, do not use beer! It's necessary for the menstruum to be high in alcohol, so as to preserve the tincture.

2.   To make the menstruum, mix in alcohol/apple cider vinegar to a ratio of 3:1 with water and the menstruum with the thyme with a ratio of 2:1.

3.   Take 3 ounces (90grams) of alcohol/vinegar to a ratio of about 1 ounce (30 grams) of water. Then place the mix into a blender and blend. The flower now has to be chopped and ground. Then add in 2 ounces (60grams) of thyme with 4 ounces (120 grams) of menstruum.

4.   Then pour into a glass container (do not use plastic), and leave it in a dark cool place.

5.   Shake every day for the next 14 days.

6.   Strain through several layers of cheesecloth and squeeze out the essence.

7.   Leave the mix which remains to settle for 12 to 16 hours, then pour out the clear liquid from the top of the jar, which is called the decant.

8.   The decant can now be Stored in a dark glass container in a dark place which should also be cold.

When you want to take it just take out a tincture dropper and use one to two drops anywhere, three to five times daily.

This tincture will last a long time because of the preserving qualities of alcohol/vinegar.

Contraindications:

Thyme is very safe herb, and is even safe for children to take, however, in rare cases it can slow down the body's ability to create blood clots. This might increase the likelihood of bruising and may slow down bleeding, if used with medications which also have the effect of slowing down blood clotting, such as aspirin, ibuprofen and warfarin.

Elderberry extract for Flu

Eldeberry (Sambucuss nigra) belongs to the Adoxaceae family of plants and is found in temperate as well as sub-tropical regions. Elderberry has been used for hundreds of years, to treat wounds and also for respiratory infections. With elderberry it is the flowers and berries which are used medicinally, but it must be borne in mind that the berries must be cooked prior to been eaten, as in raw form they are toxic.

In a study, on the effectiveness of elderberry in treating flu, they took 64 patients, splitting them up into an elderberry group and a placebo group. They found that within 24 hours the elderberry group showed a significant improvement, in symptoms, and that within 48 hours, 60% of the elderberry group showed relief from symptoms while an incredible 28% demonstrated no symptoms whatsoever!2

Elderberry can be effective in treating in the symptoms of flu, however two things need to be borne in mind. Firstly, many people take elderberry, in order to prevent the onset of the flu, but there is no scientific evidence to back elderberry as a preventant. So it makes more sense to use other herbs to boost the immune system, such as Echinacea, for example. But the right way to use elderberry, is to take it as soon as the symptoms of flu start manifesting. Don't wait until the flu is full blown, as by then the best that the elderberry can do is to reduce the symptoms, whereas taken it at the onset can radically shorten the active time of the flu virus.

Secondly, it must be remembered that influenza is a virus, and unlike bacterial infections, there are no medical treatments which work effectively on this kind of virus. So once underway, you're looking at reduction of symptoms and viral activity time. So take elderberry as soon as symptoms arise and it will shorten the viral activity, that's the best that can be achieved when dealing with the flu!

How to take Elderberry:

Elderberry Syrup: Pre-packaged syrup can be used. Take one teaspoonful (15ml) three to four times daily, for three to four days.

Homemade Elderberry Syrup

1.   Add 2 cups of dried elderberries to 4 glasses of water and add 1 cinnamon stick, and/or 1 teaspoon of garlic powder.

2.   Boil the mixture and then simmer for 5 minutes, or until the mixture has been reduced by half its volume.

3.   Remove from the stove, mix the berry solution with a large spoon or ladle, then strain the mixture.

4.   This syrup can be used as is, or if you want to add flavour then add in some honey, gently heating the syrup/honey mixture for a couple of minutes(but not boiling), then take the mixture and pour it into a glass bottle.

Contraindications:

•   Immunosuppressant's can have a decreased effect, if combined with elderberry. Immunosuppressant's are usually used to help organ rejection, as in the case of for heart and kidney transplant patients; also glucocorticoids, which are used to treat inflammatory conditions such as arthritis. For patients on immunosuppressant's are best advised to stay away from elderberry.

Other Common Cold and Flu Natural Remedies

The subject of old and flu treatments cannot be completed without a brief look at some common herbal treatments, namely garlic, honey and ginger root.

Garlic

Garlic is rich in vitamin B6, vitamin C, manganese and antioxidants. It is also known for its antibacterial and antiviral properties, meaning that garlic can both reduce the duration and intensity of a cold. It has been proven clinically to both prevent the onset of cold as well as reducing the length and severity of cold symptoms, once a cold is active.[3] How garlic manages to do so well against a virus (the common cold is a virus and virus's tend to be very difficult to either prevent or cure, usually they have to be endured), is still something of a mystery, but a substance called 'allicin' has been noted as one compound which alleviates nasal inflammation.

How to take garlic

Cooked garlic and Raw Garlic: Garlic is usually used as an additive to add taste to food. In the process it also helps to prevent the concurrence for the common cold. However, in cooked form it is relatively ineffective, due to the effect of cooking. In raw form it is much more powerful, but it is also quite strong in taste, so usually only small amounts are taken raw. Also, in raw form it can have quite an acidic effect on the stomach.

Capsule Form: Capsules are very easy to take, they are more effective than cooked garlic and there are no issues regarding taste or stomach ache. One or two garlic capsules, taken daily, will greatly reduce the onset of the cold virus.

In summary, garlic is extremely safe and can also be quite tasty, when combined with food. Furthermore in small daily doses, it can help prevent the onset of the common cold. In the case of a cold common on, take a large dose of garlic multiple times a day, and more than likely the cold will run its course, within a couple of days rather than the usual week or so that it usually takes.

A bottle of honey is to be found in most kitchen cupboards around the world today; it's tasty and supposedly nutritious but also it has a litany of health effects, and one of those health effects relates to cold and flu symptoms.

Honey contains antioxidants, antimicrobial and antibacterial properties which help, the body to fight off viruses, bacteria and fungus. It also boosts the immune system, which reduces the likelihood of developing a cold in the first place, and of course honey will also sooth sore throats.

In a study of microbial activity and honey, they found that at concentrations of 50%, honey was effective at inhibiting Pseudomonas aeruginosa and Escherichia. Simply put, a high concentration of natural honey is effective both at preventing and treating bacterial infection. 4 Not only is honey a good way to treat bacterial infection, but also it is helpful for people who are suffering from the common cold virus. In one study, on coughing in children at night - time, they found that children who took honey before bedtime had a significant relief from coughing symptoms, when compared with children who did not take honey, suggesting that honey helps to relief the symptoms of cough and sore throat.5

How to Take Honey:

We all know how to take honey, simply open the jar and take a tablespoon and swallow it. But also we have to bear in mind the type of honey been taking, as a great many cheap honey's are virtually useless, as their purity levels are low. As a rule of thumb, the darker the honey the better the quality, and also organic is usually better than processed, but that also depends upon whether the organic honey has been made to high standards are not. It's a good idea to do some research, in your area, and see what the best honey which you can afford is.

Lemon, Ginger and Honey Tea

Ingredients:

- Two lemons

- Two pieces of fresh ginger

- Raw honey

- Glass jar

Procedure:

1. Slice the ginger and the lemons.

2. Place the slice in a glass jar.

3. Pour in the honey until the jar is full.

4. Place a wax sheet over the lid and close the lead tight so as to get a good seal.

5. Store in the refrigerator. Over time the solution will meld into a jelly like substance.

6. Whenever required, take out two or three tablespoons including some ginger and lemon, mix into boiling water and steep for five minutes, filter and then drink.

Contraindications:

Honey, as we all know is really safe; however it should not be given to children under one year of age, for fear of botulism which might take place via tiny pieces of dust mixed in with the honey during manufacture. This is fine, for even small kids, to take honey but for babies it is potentially harmful and should be avoided.

Like honey ginger is found in a great many homes across the world. Some prefer it as a powder or as a paste, while others like to stick to raw ginger. Whichever way you look at it, ginger is a very flexible herb and an excellent culinary herb at that. But also like honey it contains a great many medicinal properties which are not well known.

Ginger is an antiviral, it is an antiseptic and has anti-inflammatory properties, it is an antihistamine and a decongestant, and it is a pain inhibitor and a mild sedative. Also, it contains chemical called sesquiterpenes, which help to target rhinoviruses, and has been proven effectively in clinical trials.6

How to take Ginger:

Ginger is extremely common and often comes as a powder or in paste form, but by far the most potent form of ginger as a raw herb. Ginger can easily be added to foods and cooked, and probably one of the most effective and nice tasting ways to take ginger is as a tea infusion.

How to make Ginger Tea

1.   Pour the required number of teacups of water into a pan and boil.

2.   Add four slice of ginger per cup of water and simmer for five minutes.

3.   Strain and serve.

How to make Indian Styled Ginger Tea

The Indian people love tea and tea variations and one of them is ginger tea. In the case of India they like to make a regular tea, mixed with water and milk and simply add in ginger to taste.

1.   Place water/ milk in a saucepan (50% water and 50% milk mix) and mix one teaspoon of regular tea leaves per cup of tea, also add sugar as required, usually one teaspoon per cup.

2.   Add in the slices of ginger at the rate of four slices per cup.

3.   Bring to the boil.

4.   Lower the temperature and simmer for several minutes.

5.   Boil again and lower the temperature three times in a row, in quick succession: boil – cool, boil – cool, boil-cool.

6.   Then serve via a tea strainer, so as to filter out the ginger and the tea leaves.

Regarding frequency, ginger can be taken any time, a good rule of thumb been three times daily, but do try to source raw ginger and either use it for cooking or for tea, rather than the pastes or powers as these have been processed and will certainly be less effective than the raw herb.

Contraindications:

•   There is some evidence that ginger might slow blood clotting, so if taking medications, which slow blood clotting, such as 'warfarin' and 'advil', then ginger should be avoided.

•   Ginger may reduce blood sugar, so for diabetics they have to be careful taking diabetic medicine along with ginger as it may induce low blood sugar. This is of course a good thing and diabetics should take ginger, but be careful as low blood sugar is potentially dangerous as it can result in the onset of a coma if not checked.

Headaches, everybody has them from time to time, just take a headache pill and it will go away, right? But what if you don't want to take medication, or if you are continually suffering from headaches, perhaps on a daily basis, what then?

This is where natural remedies can really help, let's take a look:

Tension headaches

There are all sorts of headaches, such as frontal headache, headache on the sides of the head, headache in the occiput (back of the head), headache on the top of the head and headache throughout the head. All of these can be labelled as tension headaches. Sometimes these general headaches are dull and sometimes they are sharp, as in a splitting headache. Other than this the most famous type of headache is a migraine. What differentiates a migraine from a general headache? A migraine tends to be very intense and involves other motor activities, frequently dizziness is felt and even nausea, often the sufferer has no other choice but to lie down and wait for the migraine to pass.

Lets take a look at herbs, which treat tension headaches and then we will move onto migraines in the next section.

Kava Kava

Kava Kava has already been mentioned in the section on anxiety, and not only is it a good anti-anxiety herb, but it is also a good pain killer for headaches. Kava Kava is basically a good mental relaxant, and as such if the headaches are tension related, the distressing effect is completely cured. Kava kava is not guaranteed to cure all tension headaches, but in many cases it will help. The only way to find out is to try kava Kava, when you have your next headache, and see how it goes. If it works continue using it and if it doesn't, then stop using it. The thing to remember with headaches, is that often the causes are varied, consequently a mental de-stressor, like kava a kava will only work in some cases.

How to take Kava:

Take a look at the serving suggestions in chapter one, on anxiety, here Kava kava is covered in detail.

Valerian

Like Kava Kava, valerian is a great way to get relieve for tension headaches. And pretty much it will work well on some and not on others. If the cause of the headache is tension related, often it will bring about a relieving effect. Like kava kava, try it out and see if it works for you.

How to take Valerian:

Take a look at the serving suggestions in chapter one, on anxiety, here Valerian is covered in detail.

We have already taken a look at passionflower in chapter one, on anxiety, but also passionflower helps with headaches too. The leaves have been proven to be very effective, at treating a variety of ailments and are noted has been a good source of harmala alkaloids, such as harmaline and harmine.

Passionflower works great as a muscle relaxant, a reliever of tensions both physical and emotional and even a really good headache cure, both for tension and even migraine headaches. It is also quite a popular ingredient in sleep, pain and anxiety aids within the European Union, but not in America.

Passionflower reduces anxiety and depressive symptoms, because harmaline and harmine are Monoamine Oxidase Inhibitors (MOI's). In action they inhibit the monoamine oxidase enzyme, which in turn prevents the breakdown of monoamine neurotransmitters, which are helpful in maintaining a good mood.1

How to take Passionflower:

Passion flower can be taken as:

- Tea

- Infusion

- Liquid extracts

- Tinctures

For more details, on making passionflower tea and infusions look up chapter two or appendix one.

58

Contraindications:

- Do not take if pregnant or breastfeeding

- Do not take with sedatives (drugs which promote sleep), such as barbiturates, benzodiazepines, such as alprazolam, insomnia drugs such as 'Ambien' and tricyclic antidepressants, such as 'Elavil'.

- Do not take with blood thinners, such as clopidogrel, warfarin and aspirin.

- Do not take it with monoamine oxidase inhibitor (MAOIs), which are an old group of antidepressants.

Interestingly, the fact that passionflower has to be avoided with sleeping medication, blood thinners and MOA anti-depressants suggest that even though research is not conclusive, that passionflower is a good treatment for sleep disorder, blood thinning and as an anti-depressant!

Migraines

How do you know whether you have a general headache or a tension headache?

Check out the list below:

- Seeing stars

- Excruciating pain

- Blinding pain whereby even thinking seems to hurt

- Nausea

- Dizziness

- Pain in the temples

- Sensitivity to light and sound

- Temporary loss of vision

- Vomiting

In a nutshell, getting a migraine is like getting hit by a sledgehammer, if you have one you won't need to double guess as you will be doubled over in pain!

Sometimes general tension headaches can develop into migraines, but by and large migraines appear to be genetic in character; if you start getting migraines on a regular basis then it's probably all to do with your genes.

But what to do about it?

Well you can take medication and take rest, but thankfully there are herbs which aid in migraine relief.

The herbs mentioned in the previous section (Kava Kava, Valerian and Passionflower) can often have a beneficial effect on migraines, but what herbs definitely work well with migraines, in a significant way?

Butterbur and Feverfew

Butterbur:

75mg of butterbur a day can reduce the onset of migraines by approximately 50%!

Butterbur and Feverfew will not make a migraine go away, however, they will help to prevent it from taking place in the first place!

We have already covered Butterbur in chapter one (on anxiety, but butterbur is also a really good herb for migraine onset prevention).

In one study, on the effect of butterbur on children, they took 108 children, aged between 6 and 17 years of age, and observed that over a period of a year 77% of the participants, reported a reduction in migraine frequency by at least 50%.2

In another study on 245 participants, they divided the group into a placebo group and a group who took 75mg of Butterbur, over a period of four months. The butterbur group saw a 48% decrease in the frequency of migraine headaches. 3

How to Take Butterbur:

We have already covered butterbur in chapter three on allergies. Take a look a chapter three for butterbur dosages and contraindications.

Feverfew:

Feverfew (Tanacetum parthenium) belongs to the daisy family, and originated in south Eastern Europe but is now found thought Europe, America and Australia. Feverfew is effective at treating inflammation, and appears to relieve spasms in smooth muscle tissue, via a chemical called parthenolide. Feverfew is also an effective preventative for migraines, although scientists are not sure as to how it is that feverfew operates.

Regardless, scientific evidence does support the effectiveness of feverfew. In a 2005 study over a 16 week period, they observed that the migraine frequency decreased from 4.79 to 2.89 attacks per month! 4

How to take Feverfew:

Feverfew usually comes as either a capsule or as dried leaves. The capsule will usually be anywhere from 200mmg to 400mg, and most are standardised to have parthenolide 0.7% per capsules contents. Depending upon the quantity, per capsule, anywhere from one to three capsules can be taken per day.

If you can get your hands on feverfew dried leaves then it's easy to make a refreshing cup of tea.

How to make Feverfew Tea:

1.   Pour one cup of boiling water over one tablespoon full of dried feverfew leaves.

2.   Steep for thirty to sixty minutes.

3.   Strain and serve.

Feverfew Contraindications:

•   Medications which slow blood clotting, such as Nizoral and Halcion will not work as effectively if taken while on feverfew.

•   Pregnant ladies and breastfeeding mothers.

•   Children under two years of age.

So far we have looked at tension headaches and migraines, however there are several other types of headaches which also must be considered.

Cluster headaches

Cluster headaches are headaches which effect one side of the head, are often accompanies by a watery eye and nasal congestion, and possibly even a runny nose on one side of the face. With cluster headaches, they often come in groups or cycles, such as every day or three days in a row, followed by a week break and then another three days in a row and so on.

During an attack, often the person will feel restless and usually, unlike a migraine, they do not feel like lying down and resting.

As yet there is no known cause of cluster headaches, but they do appear to have a genetic component and they also appear to affect more men than women.

If you suffer from cluster headache it would be a good idea to get checked out by your doctor. They might be able to give some medication to help, plus they can run some tests and make sure that it's just a headache and nothing more complex. After all, we are talking about our heads here and in particular our brain. There are many potential candidates for one sided headaches, which need to be tested for and eliminated, such as high blood pressure, arterial congestion and even brain tumour. Don't start worrying, but do check these things out and make sure that it's just a cluster headache which you are dealing with.

If a cluster headache has been diagnosed, do take the required medicine. If you would like to try out a natural remedy then try out Kudzu.

Kudzu, otherwise known as Japanese Arrowroot, belongs to the genus Pueraria. They are climbing vines, which come from Asia, Southeast Asia and some of the Pacific Islands.

In a study on the effectiveness of Kudzu, as a cure for cluster headaches, they discover that 69% of the participants, who took kudzu, experienced decreased intensity of the attacks and 31% experienced decreased duration, of the attacks![5]

How to take Kudzu:

Kudzu usually comes in capsule form, with dosage varying anywhere from 1 to 12 grams per day. Most academic studies stick to a small dose of around 900mg a day, so it is better to start on a low dose and increase as needs be. Taking kudzu at a high dosage for a long time may have some toxic effects.

Kudzu Contraindications:

•   Do not take if breastfeeding or pregnant.

•   Kudzu might slow down blood clotting and if used alongside blood clotting medication, it may make the medication less effective.

•   Kudzu lowers blood pressure and may result in low blood pressure episodes for people who are on high blood pressure medication.

- Kudzu might be hazardous to the lover and should not be used by liver patients.

The sinuses are cavities in the skull, in the forehead, cheeks and over the bridge of the nose. The role of the sinuses is twofold. Firstly, they modulate the temperature of the air coming into the body, so that the lungs receive air which is warm enough to function properly, and secondly they filter out bacteria, virus and funguses. When the sinuses are working well, you wouldn't even know that they exist, however, when they become enflamed, lots of health conditions can kick off, and one of these is the infamous sinus headache.

Sinus headaches usually involve a deep ache behind the cheekbones, which worsens with sudden movement. Often the head will feel heavy and a dull ache will be found in the forehead, and behind the eyes, and a runny nose sometimes accompanies this type of headache.

There are many medications for sinusitis, however, most sinus sufferer's find that they only give temporary relief, and that they have to grin and bear their sinusitis and sinus headaches. However, there are many things which can be done.

Cast your mind back to chapter three (on allergies), where we spoke about the herbs quercetin, butterbur and stinging nettle. Each of these are really good naturally anti-histamines, and these can often help because they reduce the allergic reaction, which inflamed the sinuses in the first place.

Also, let's not forget Feverfew. Feverfew as well as treating migraines has also been found to work well on sinus headaches.

Another useful herb is Eucalyptus. Eucalyptus oil is really famous for its many beneficial effects. One of these effects is an improvement in sinus headaches and this is because of cieneole, which is very effective at treating sinusitis. 6

How to take Eucalyptus Oil

Eucalyptus is very flexible and can be taken in several ways, which are:

Stream Inhalation: Here you add several drops of Eucalyptus oil to a large bowl of boiled water, place a towel over your head and breathe in deeply. This is one of the most satisfying ways to take this oil as relief is instantaneous and deeply satisfying.

Dilution and Application: This is a little more direct than steam inhalation, it can be effective, and the good thing is that it is less cumbersome than steam inhalation, but some people find it irritating, so try it out and see how it works for you.

Add a few drop of Eucalyptus oil in with non-irritating oil, and then rub it directly onto the facial area. In diluted form Eucalyptus can be really potent with little or no irritation.

Direct Application: Is for people who have very insensitive skin. This is really easy, simply rub the oil into the sensitive area, that's it.

Eucalyptus Contraindications:

• Eucalyptus might reduce blood sugar, consequently when combined with diabetic medicine low blood sugar may result. This also indicates that Eucalyptus is good for lowering blood sugar levels!

Other Considerations for Headaches

We have covered a variety of headaches, in this chapter. One thing to bear in mind, about headaches, is that there are a wide variety of causes and each one takes a different approach. However, on another level, some generalities apply.

For example, to some degree all headaches are caused by tension, so all the herbs used for migraines, cluster and sinusitis can be assisted by Passionflower, Valerian and Kava. So focus on a base of relaxing anti-tension herbs and then use specific herbs for the specific type of headache so as to effectively treat that particular headache.

Chapter Six – Stomach

Apple cider vinegar

Apple cider vinegar is a type of vinegar made from cider or apple and is a base.

Base's have a high pH whereas acids have a low pH. Both acids and base's appear acidic in nature as in they can produce a burning sensation, in some cases, but their action is very different As a rule of thumb because of the foods which we presently eat, most people are too acidic, which results in all sorts of aches and pains. Base's frequently help to bring the body back to balance, hence one of the chief benefits of Apple Cider Vinegar (ACV) is in how it helps to treat arthritic conditions, which are brought upon via the production of uric acid deposits in the joints. Also, when the body's pH is balanced, it appears less likely for it to develop cancerous growths, as tumours are more likely to grow in an acidic environment.

Many other benefits are to be had with ACV which includes heart health, weight loss, and diabetic benefits. But another benefit relates to the stomach. For a start ACV is an effective antimicrobial and antibacterial1, which in itself can help to protect the body from stomach infections and also to treat them when they arise.

Also, apple cider vinegar appears to have a good effect on balancing stomach acids, and may well prove to be more effective than antacids, at doing this. There is anecdotal evidence for this, rather than scientific, but it appears to be that stomach acid problems come about possibly from an imbalance, rather than from over acidity. Either way imbibing apple cider vinegar, which is a base, seems to have a good effect on upset stomachs, in many cases.

Also, as noted above, ACV appears to have all round health benefits and can be seen as an overall tonic for the body.

How to take Apple Cider Vinegar:

Simply add one teaspoon of Apple Cider Vinegar to one 250ml glass of water and drink it. Yes it is sour, just drink it quickly and move on. As a tonic, once a day is good, for stomach upsets it could be taken when the stomach is upset and can be taken up to three times a day without side effects (remember too much base is just as bad for you as too much acid).

To sum up ACV, it's worth trying out next time you have an upset stomach. However, more importantly, it is a superb tonic which will vivify your health and help prevent stomach upsets and other health problems from kicking off on the first place.

Apple Cider Vinegar Contraindications:

•   It can reduce potassium levels in the body are taken in excess.

•   Diuretics lower potassium levels and if combined with Apple Cider Vinegar will reduce potassium to an even greater degree, which could be very dangerous.

•   Large amounts of insulin may reduce potassium levels and if taken with Apple Cider Vinegar, may once again be bad for the body.

Lemon juice has so many beneficial properties. First of all lemon juice, while it is acidic, it breaks down into a base once ingested into the body, which in turn is a really good way to help alkalinise the body. The human body should be alkaline, meaning its pH should be around pH 7.35 – 7.45 or so. However, most of us are acidic, because of the foods which we eat. So drinking some lemon juice every day is a great health tonic.

It's also a good way to start the day, on an empty stomach about half an hour prior to breakfast as it triggers the stomach into releasing hydrochloric acid, while also increasing bile production from the liver, which in turn aids digestion. This way when we eat our food the stomach immediately works on digesting it. This helps digestion, but also it triggers the metabolism which can aid with weight loss.

From a stomach ache point of view, lemon juice helps because it makes the stomach produce more acid, which helps to balance stomach. Also, just like Apple Cider Vinegar it's a base, and so it helps to regulate the pH of the body, which in turn reduces the likelihood of stomach problems in the first place.

How to take Lemon juice:

Lemon juice is really acidic in flavour, so it's impossible to take in pure form. However, when mixed with some water and a little sugar, it is tasty, refreshing, good for rehydration and general health.

A tasty way to take lemon juice is as follows:

1.   Add one teaspoon of lemon juice to a 200ml glass of water.

2.   Add a teaspoon of honey.

71

3.   Mix well and drink.

For something a little more exotic try:

1.   Take a 200ml glass of water and add one teaspoon of lemon juice.

2.   Add a teaspoon of honey, one teaspoon of ginger juice and a pinch of black pepper.

3.   Mix well and drink.

Sourcing Lemon Juice:

Lemon juice can be bought but also it can be homemade and is really easy to do. Simply take 20 small lemons or five big ones, cut squeeze and juice. Then filter and pour into a glass jar and store in the refrigerator. This way it can be stored for up to about two months.

Note:

While both Apple Cider Vinegar and lemon juice, are acidic in effect (even though ACV is a base and lemon juice is an acid which breaks down into a base within the body), but in action they are acidic. Consequently they can damage enamel in the teeth, so make sure you rinse your mouth with water after wards, so as to protect the teeth.

Aloe Vera is a succulent plant and is widely used for cosmetics as well as in many complimentary health products. Aloe vera is one of the oldest and most effective plants, which can be used to treat a wide range of health problems such as detoxing the body, alkalising the body, it enhances cardiovascular health, it benefits the skin and it helps with weight loss.

Regarding the stomach, aloe vera helps in a couple of ways. First of all just like apple cider vinegar and Lemon juice, it helps to alkalinise the body which brings about balance, but also secondly it aids digestion. Since indigestion is often a cause of stomach ache, anything which aids digestion is good. Aloe vera also helps the intestinal tract, relieving constipation which in turn often takes pressure of off the stomach, which is often overwhelmed if intestinal blockage is preventing food from exiting the stomachs.Even peptic ulcers appear to improve, once treated with aloe vera. In a study of 18 peptic ulcer patients, 17 of them recovered when they took Aloe Vera gel emulsion!2

How to take Aloe Vera Juice:

Aloe vera can be taken in 40-5ml doses up to 3 times a day.

Chapter 7 – Nausea

Closely related to stomach ailments and imbalances is nausea. From time to time everyone sufferers from nausea, but what can we do about it other than taking allopathic medications?

Well let's take a look:

Ginger

Ginger is a wonderful herb. It is fantastic for food preparation and also it is a great herbal therapy. We have already looked at it in detail in chapter four (colds and flu's) and it's worth noting that it also helps to relieve stomach ache.

Why ginger works so effectively, is still unknown but its efficacy has been scientifically proven. In a study on 70 mothers suffering from morning sickness, they were split into two groups, a placebo group and a ginger group, over a 5 month period. The ginger group were given 1g of oral ginger per day. By the end of the study 28 out of the 32 participants, who took ginger, had improvement in their nausea symtpoms.[1]

The nice thing with ginger is that it's a really safe herbs and it can even be taking by pregnant mothers, which is really great. For consumption information and contraindications check out the ginger section in chapter four.

Peppermint (Mentha piperita, which is also known as M. balsamea Wild) belongs to the mint family and has long been used as a herbal home remedy.

Peppermint has a calming and numbing effect, which helps to settle down an upset stomach. Because it relaxes the stomach muscles, this allows the stomach to release bile, which breaks down fats and helps to move the food out of the stomach. Also, in a study on the effects of peppermint, on post-operative nausea, found a statistically notable difference on the post-operative patients who used Peppermint versus the ones who did't.[2]

Furthermore, peppermint is effective at treating irritable bowel syndrome (IBS), as it relaxes the intestinal walls. Overall peppermint is a great gastrointestinal muscle relaxant, which means it can be good for stomach aches, constipation and nausea.

How to take Peppermint:

Peppermint Tea

Peppermint tea is the most famous, and tasty way, to take Peppermint. Peppermint tea is widely available at health food shops and even supermarkets. You can also make your own Peppermint tea, as follows:

1.   Boil water.

2.   Place peppermint leaves or extract in a cup of tea pot and pour water.

3.   Leave to soak for about five minutes.

4.   Filter and drink.

Peppermint Oil: Peppermint can also be taken in oil form:

1.   Wash the peppermint leaves and chop them.

2.   Place them in a jar with carrier oil, such as olive oil, for instance. Seal the jar, ideally with wax paper on the lid and leave to soak for 24 hours.

3.   Strain the oil and add additional peppermint leaves and olive oil reseal and leave for another 24 hours.

4.   Repeat every day for 5 days.

5.   Finally remove the peppermint leaves and strain the oil into a glass container.

Peppermint Capsules: Another approach is to take peppermint capsules, at the rate of 1 to 3 per day.

Peppermint Contraindications:

•   It interacts badly with Cyclosporine (Neoral, Sandimmune).

•   Medications which are changed by the liver such as (Cytochrome P450 1A2 (CYP1A2) substrates) and (Cytochrome P450 2C19 (CYP2C19) substrates) interacts with Peppermint, which might result in a slower absorption times in these medicines.

•   Other medications will also suffer from decreased absorption times such as Ibuprofen, Nizoral and Halcion, for example.

Good old lemon, which we have already covered in chapter six (on stomach ache) as well as throughout the book, in various herbal concoctions, so it's no surprise to find that lemon is also good for treating nausea.

In a study, on treating pregnant ladies suffering from morning sickness, they took 100 pregnant women and split them into two groups. One group inhaled lemon essential oil while the other group was inhaling a placebo. Out of the lemon essential oil group, they saw a significant reduction in morning sickness symptoms, within several days of initiating the lemon essential oil inhalation treatment![3] Also, the nausea and vomiting intensity in the second and fourth days in the intervention group were also significantly lower than the control group! [3]

How to take Lemon

Lemon water: Simply squeeze a lemon, filter it and add it to some water and sugar to taste.

Lemon Oil: Lemon essential oil can be bought at most health food stores and it is easy take. Simply pour a few drops on a handkerchief and sniff it whoever you feel nauseas. This is ideal for pregnant women suffering from morning sickness and people in general who are feeling nausea yet they are in public and who don't want to make a scene.

Cloves are famous for their toothache relieving benefits, but they are also helpful at treating the symptoms of nausea. Cloves possess anti-inflammatory properties which help to relax the muscles of the stomach, which in turn helps to relieve nausea.

How to take Cloves:

Clove Tea: Simply boil 250ml of water and add 1 tsp. of clove powder (or 4 clove pods) to it, filter and drink.

Cloves and Honey: Add a small amount of ground and roasted clove pods to 1 tsp. of honey, mix and drink up to 4 times a day.

Clove Oil Inhalation: Simply sprinkle a few drops of clove oil onto your pillow at night, or on your handkerchief during the day. This is ideal for pregnant ladies suffering from morning sickness and busy people who are worried about making a scene in public.

Cloves Contraindications:

• Medications which slow clotting Anticoagulant / Antiplatelet drugs) work more slowly when combined with cloves, for example Aspirin, Ibuprofen and Warfarin.

Cumin

Cumin is a flowering plant, which belongs to the Apiaceous family and is a native of the Eastern Mediterranean and India, and is now widely used as a condiment to the food making process. Cumin is also quite famous, for its many health benefits which includes immunity boosting, improving digestion, preventing cancer, improving diabetic symtpoms,improving insomnia, improving respiratory disorders and of course as a treatment for nausea.

How to take Cumin

Cumin Tea: Boil 250ml of water and then add the cloves, and leave it to steep for ten minutes. Filter out the cumin seeds and drink.

Chewing Cumin: Chew one teaspoon of dry roasted cumin seeds.

Cumin Contraindications:

• Medications which slow clotting Anticoagulant / Antiplatelet drugs) work more slowly when combined with cloves, for example Aspirin,Ibuproven and Warfarin.

Fennel

Fennel is a florin plant of the carrot family and is quite famous as a tea. However, Fennel also has a lot of really good health befits which includes anaemia, blood pressure, constipation, indigestion, flatulence, heart disease, and cancer, and of course nausea.

Scientists are not quite sure why fennel is so effective but it does contain Anethole, a phytoestrogen, which is likely the active compound. Anethole appears to help the expulsion of gas, from the stomach, as well as acting as a muscle relaxant which helps the stomach to relax along with the intestinal tract.

How to take Fennel

Fennel Tea: Fennel tea is a popular item in most health food stores. But it can also be easily be made at home by boiling water, mixing in some fennel seeds and stepping for 10 minutes, then filtering and drinking.

Chewing Fennel Seeds: Simply take one teaspoon of fennel seeds and chew them slowly.

For people, who are prone to nausea, it is a good idea to take fennel seeds after meals, otherwise fennel can be taken upto four times a day, as necessary.

Fennel Contraindications:

- Birth control pills if combined with fennel might lose some of their potency.

- The antibiotic Ciprofloxacin (Cipro) will lose some of its potency when mixed with fennel.

- Tamoxifen (Nolvadex) is used to treat and prevent certsin types of cancer. It might become less effective if combined with fennel.

While there is a lot of research, on the benefits of herbs on skin conditions, by and large most of this research is sponsored by skin care companies, hence it is difficult to know exactly which herb is best and why. One thing to realise though, is that often when skin care companies advertise their product and boast all sort of clinical evidence for this product, that often it's not true!

So should we use skin creams which are commercially available?

Well yes, certainly if they are effective, but don't just sign up because of the advertising. Meanwhile let's take a look at some popular herbs, which have anecdotally been proven to be effective.

Baking Soda

Baking soda is as old as the hills and it's very effective and easy to take. Baking soda has great skin cleansing properties, plus it eliminates breakouts of acne, while reducing skin inflammation and exfoliating at the same time.

How to take Baking Soda:

Baking Soda mixed with Cleanser: When trying out baking soda, for the first time, this is a good idea, as it is a way for you to assess its effectiveness and make sure that you do not have a bad reaction to it.

1.   Simply add half a teaspoon of baking soda to your cleanser, mix it and then message into the skin.

2.   Wash off.

3.   Immediately rub in moisturiser

Face Mask: Face masks are a great way to reduce inflammation and redness of the skin.

1.   Cleanse the face with a gentle cleanser.

2.   Mix 2 teaspoons of baking soda with water and make a paste.

3.   Apply to the skin and leave it for 15 minutes. If it stings a little then ok, if it is too irritating then take it off. Also, do try the cleanser approach first, so to assess for any allergic reactions. Also, the first time you put on the baking soda mask, just try it for a few minutes, wash it off and check for any reactions, always be careful when applying anything to your skin for the first time.

4.   Wash off and apply moisturiser.

Cleansing Spots: Because baking soda is such a good anti-inflammatory, it is very good at spot reduction. Also this particular approach is very useful for anyone who has very sensitive skin, whereby the cleanser and mask approach is possible to irritating.

1.   Mix a little bit of baking soda and water and apply directly to a pimple, cyst or inflamed area.

2.   Leave on for 20 minutes.

3.   Let it harden.

4.   Then remove and apply some moisturiser.

Apple Cider Vinegar

We already came across apple cider vinegar in chapter six (on stomach ache). It's a great product which treats so many conditions and can generally be considered as a health tonic. We would all benefit from drinking a tablespoon of apple cider vinegar mixed with a glass of water, everyday.

Anyway moving onto skin conditions, apple cider vinegar is a strong antibacterial and anti-fungal. Also Apple Cider Vinegar is good for age spots, it a good cleanser and it helps relieve symptoms for acne.

How it use Apple Cider Vinegar

Note: Never apply undiluted to the skin and Apple Cider Vinegar is a strong base!

Apple Cider Vinegar Toner: Mix Apple Cider Vinegar to water at the ratio of 50:50.

More Exotic Toner: Mix Apple Cider Vinegar with green tea or aloe Vera gel or witch hazel.

Direct Application: Mix ACV with water and soak a cotton bud. Then rub on the skin in affected areas.

Comparing an ointment with 5% tea tree oil versus a standard 5% benzoyl peroxide lotion, the scientists discovered that each was equally effective at reducing skin inflammation

Tea tree oil is an essential oil, which has a marvellous effect on skin conditions such as mouth ulcers, abscesses, boils, impetigo, dandruff, psoriasis, thrush, septic wounds, carbuncles, pus-filled infections, ringworm and of course acne.

In a study of 124 acne patients, they compared an ointment with 5% tea tree oil versus a standard 5% benzoyl peroxide lotion. Comparing the two, the scientists discovered that each was equally effective at reducing skin inflammation, with two exceptions. Firstly the benzoyl peroxide lotion was quicker to act and that secondly the tea tree oil had far fewer side effects.[1]

How to use Tea Tree Oil

Cleanser and Moisturizer: Simply add a few drops of tea tree oil in with your cleanser or moisturiser.

Facial Scrub:

1. Mix half a cup of sugar with 1 tbsp. of honey, ¼ cup of sesame or olive oil with 10 drops of tea tree oil in a small bowl.

2. Gently scrub the face for 5 minutes.

3. Rinse off with Luke warm water and dry.

Facial masks:

Here are three variations:

1.   Take 2 tbsp. of green clay powder and mix in 3 to 4 drops of tea tree oil. Add water and mix so as to form a paste. Apply onto the face and leave it for 20 minutes. Rinse with lukewarm water and dry.

2.   Mix 1 tsp. of jojoba oil with 3 drops of tea tree oil and add in a finely chopped tomato. Mix into a puree and apply on as a face mask. Leave for 20 minutes then use some arm water to wash it off.

3.   Take a ¼ cup of plain yoghurt and add in 5 drop soft tea tree oil. Apply directly to the face and leave for 20 minutes. Wash off with lukewarm water and dry.

Spot Treatment:

1.   Take a few drops of aloe vera gel and add in a couple of drops of oil into it. If you don't have aloe vera simply use honey in its place.

2.   Apply mixture directly to pimple, or area of sensitive skin.

Apply to Pimples Directly:

1.   Add a couple of drop soft tea tree oil to a cotton bud.

2.   Dab the affected area with the cotton bud.

Herbs for Skin Contraindications:

Are herbs safe to use on our skin?

The answer to this question is yes. In general herbs are far gentler on the skin than artificially made lotions. Also, many artificial lotions use these herbs in their formulations. So why spend a lot of money on a cream, consisting largely of herbs and fillers, when you can use the herbs themselves, which are cheaper and gentler in their effect on our skin!

Furthermore, for those of us who have to use medications on our skin, often it is better to try out the herbs first, as they often work out well without all the nasty side effects.

So in general herbs are a great option for skin care.

However, our skin is the most sensitive organ of our bodies and great care needs to be taken. Even a herb can result in an allergic reaction, so prior to trying out a herbal lotion or application, be careful and spot check the herb. Which means to try out a small amount on one little piece of skin, leave for 5 minutes and see if any allergic reactions are taking place. If there is a reaction, wash it off immediately and don't use it again. If there is no reaction, then try out one of the more gently options, such as using the herb for direct application, whereby a little bit of the herb is put onto a cotton bud and applied directly. If that goes ok, then next time consider maybe using it mixed in with a cleanser. If that goes ok then try a facial mask.

Think of it this way, direct application results in a second or two second exposure to the herb, whereas a facial mask, for example, represents a 20 minute exposure. So for safety sake, start with minimal exposure and work upward, and this applies to each and every herb. This is general advice for everybody, but its special advice for those who are suffering from sensitive skin and acute skin conditions to be extra careful.

Avocado Soybean Unsaponifiables (ASU)

ASU is a natural vegetable extract, which is made from 1/3 avocado oil and 2/3 soybean oil. In action ASU blocks the pro-inflammatory chemicals, prevents deterioration in the synovial cells (which are the cells which line the joints) and may even help to regenerate connective tissue. In a study in 2003, it was noted that ASU inhibited the breakdown of cartilage and even helped to repair the cartilage, to some degree.[1] In a 2008 study, they saw evidence of improved symptoms, of hip and knee arthritis, as well as a reduced or even eliminated use of non-steroidal anti-inflammatory drugs (NDAIDS).[2]

How to take ASU: ASu comes in capsules and up to 300mg can be taken a day.

ASU Contraindications:

•   Avocado interacts with warfarin thus reducing its ability to prevent clotting.

•   Monoamine Oxidase Inhibitors (MAOI's) anti-depressants are inhibited by soya and may lose some effectiveness

Black currant seed oil is obtained from the seeds of the black currant. These seeds contain 15% to 20% gamma-linolenic acid (GLA). GLA lowers joint pain, reduces stiffness and swelling which is associated with rheumatoid arthritis. In a study of 56 patients, who took 2.8 grams a day of GLA, they noticed a significant improvement in their arthritis conditions. They noticed an improvement in grip strength within six months and noted a continued improvement in arthritic conditions, over the period of one year.

Interestingly GLA, even though it is fairly slow to act and requires daily dosing, when GLA is combined with evening primrose oil and fish oil (Efamol), that in many cases regular arthritic medications could be stopped altogether!3

How to take Black Currant Oil:

GLA makes up approximately 1/5th of black currant seed oil, so in order to get 2.8g's requires at least 5 times that amount of black currant seed oil. The easiest way to get this is via capsules, which are widely available in health food stores. Dosing been anywhere from 360mg to 3000mg per day.

Black Currant Oil Contraindications:

• GLA interacts with anticoagulants and antiplatelet drugs, thus reducing their effectiveness.

• Phenothiazine's interact with GLA, and the chance of seizures may increase if the two are combined.

Evening primrose is quite a famous medicinal plant. It helps many conditions including alzheimer's, multiple sclerosis, skin disorders and as a preventative for diabetic nerve damage, to mention but a few. Evening primrose is a must have for anyone who is interested in using herbal remedies. Also, just like black currants it contains lots of GLA, approximately 7% to 10%. Less than that of black currant, but still a significant amount, as in enough to help reduce many arthritic conditions, especially when used alongside black currant.

How to take Evening Primrose

Capsules: Take from 540mg up to 2.8g per day split into 5 doses.

Evening Primrose Oil Contraindications:

•   Can cause bloating in some cases.

•   GLA interacts with anticoagulants and antiplatelet drugs, thus reducing their effectiveness.

•   It may react with medications during surgery.

•   Phenothiazine's interact with GLA, and the chance of seizures may increase if the two are combined.

Fish oil capsules contain the oil from cold water fish such as salmon, mackerel, herring, tuna, cod and halibut.

Fish oils are high in omega-3 fatty acids (including EPA and DHA), which block cytokines and prostaglandins, thus reducing inflammation. Also, EPA and DHA is converted into anti-inflammatory substances called resolvin, which once again helps to reduce inflammation. Furthermore, fish oil reduces triglyceride (bad cholesterol), which in turn helps to reduce blood pressure and protects the heart in the process.

In a study of 40 rheumatoid arthritic patients, over 14 weeks, they noted that the participants, who took fish oil, saw a subjective alleviation in rheumatoid arthritis symptoms, as well as a reduction in neutrophil leukotriene B4 production, thus reducing inflammation.4

How to take Fish Oil

Eating Fish: Ideally, the average person requires a 3 ounce (85gs) serving of fish twice a week. For those who don't want to eat fish they can take capsules or tablets instead.

Fish oil can also be taken as capsules, soft gels, chewable or in liquid form. To treat Rheumatoid arthritis, take capsules which contain at least 30% EPA/DHA. Take 2.8g's of EPA and 2g's of DHA, per day.

Fish Oil Contraindications:

*   Do not take while on birth control pills.

92

- Fish oil sometimes interacts badly with high pressure medications such as Capote, Vaster and Norvasc.

- Orlistat (a weight loss pill), blocks absorption of triglycerides which may also prevent the effective absorption of fresh oil.

There are some really great herbal remedies, which treat hypertension. It must also be noted that hypertension is an imbalance, and as long as the cardiovascular system is healthy, it should be possible to address high blood pressure naturally, over time.

Note: In this chapter some research on the effectiveness of herbs is noted. To provide you with a little frame of reference, to help understand the research better, a quick overview of blood pressure readings follows.

Clinical researchers, into high blood pressure focus on the two major markers of high blood pressure. These are called systolic and diastolic. Systolic refers to the pressure in the arteries, as blood leaves the heart, whereas diastolic blood pressure refers to the pressure of blood, on its way back to the heart. Ideally a person should be in the range of 80 diastolic and 120 systolic. The systolic will be higher because the blood is coming from the heart. So this reading is referred to as 120/80, which we call as 120 over 80. Once this figure reaches 90/140, we are entering into high blood pressure and once it reaches 150/100 it is full blown high blood pressure.

While it is good to see a drop in both diastolic and systolic blood pressure levels, when research material is mentioned, the focus in this chapter is mainly upon diastolic levels (the lower level of the two, as the blood heads back towards the heart), because this is seen as the most relevant indicator of blood pressure. Basically the systolic will fluctuate a lot due to activity, for example exercise will raise the systolic, whereas the diastolic should remain fairly constant.

Cinnamon

Cinnamon is a spice which comes from the inner bark of several trees, which belong to the genus Cinnamomum, and is most popular as a food condiment.

Cinnamon, also has many health benefits which includes improved blood sugar control, irritable bowel syndrome (IBS) symptoms, arthritic symptoms, memory improver and antibacterial/antimicrobial, to name but a few.

Cinnamon also works well as a high blood pressure treatment. In a study of 58 type 2 diabetic patients, which were split into a placebo group and a cinnamon group, the placebo group saw a drop in their diastolic blood pressure, from an average of 85.2 to 80.2, which is a considerable decrease.1 In another study, on the effect of cinnamon, on 44 diabetic patients, discovered the levels of fasting blood glucose, HbA1c levels, triglycerides, bodyweight, BMI as well as body fat mass, decreased significantly compared to baseline.2

How to take Cinnamon:

Around 2g a day of Cinnamon, is enough to produce a good effect, and a maximum of around 4g a day can be taken, as high does can produce toxicity.

Cinnamon in Food: Cinnamon can easily be added to food in the cooking process.

Cinnamon Capsules: Cinnamon can be taken in capsule form.

Cinnamon Tea: Cinnamon can also be taken as a tea.

1.   Add water to a stick of Ceylon cinnamon.

2.   Boil slowly so as to release the cinnamon from the stick.

3.   Eventually the water should turn a mild brown colour, this should take about 15 minutes.

4.   Leave it to sit for 15 to 20 minutes, so as to settle down. You will know it is ready when the colour suddenly changes from brown to a red colour.

Cinnamon Contraindications:

•   Cinnamon reduces blood sugar levels. If diabetic, measure your blood sugar so as to make sure that it's not running too low, as when can among is combined with diabetic medicines it can result in low blood sugar levels.

•   Hepatic drugs (drugs which are harmful to the liver) interact badly when combined with cinnamon.

•   Taking large doses of cinnamon, for people who are suffering from liver disease might also be toxic to the liver.

Garlic

In a meta-analysis over a 52 year period, the scientists noted that garlic was effective at making significant reductions in blood pressure levels!!!

We have already looked at garlic in chapter four, on treating cold and flu's, but garlic has also be proven to help reduce blood pressure levels. In a meta-analysis (a broad overview study of many previous academic studies) of 25 studies between 1955 and 2007, revealed that the mean (average over a lot of data) levels of diastolic blood pressure had dropped 7.3+/-1.5mg. In plain English this means that over a wide range of studies, across a 52 year period, that on average participants who took garlic saw a substantial drop in diastolic blood pressure levels!3

Garlic appears to be an effective treatment, for high blood pressure, thanks to a compound known as allicin. We've already seen how allicin helps to treat the common cold, but also it is a good way to treat high blood pressure, and has been proven to do so in clinical trials.4

How to take Garlic and Contraindications:

We have already covered this in detail in chapter 4, just take a look, as there are lots of ways to take garlic.

Garlic Doses for Hypertension:

In a study, which appeared in the Pakistan Journal of Pharmaceutical Sciences, on garlic dosing for hypertensive patients, using doses varying from 300, 600, 900, 1200 or 1500 milligrams of garlic per day, their research demonstrated that each dose became increasingly effective. In other words 300mg is effective, but 900mg is more effective and 1500mg is even more effective. So the good news is that any amount of garlic, will help to reduce blood pressure levels but a higher amount, will do better.

Aiming for a higher amount, of say 1500mg a day will make a significant improvement. In the study, over 24 weeks the average systolic levels were at

97

145mg +/-0.706 in week zero and this decreased down to 138.6mg +/-0.850 by week 24. So this is a big drop of 9.5%, which is substantial. Although it needs to be noted, as tends to be the case with herbs, the effect takes time. Whereas allopathic medicine will work in hours, herbs can work well in days and weeks, but if taken daily the effects can be sustained and often with little or no negative side effects!

Ginger

Ginger works the same way as a calcium channel blocker hypertensive medication!

Ginger like garlic works great at treating cold and flu's, but also like garlic it helps to reduce high blood pressure. In a study on the action of ginger, on high blood pressure, they noted that ginger lowers blood pressure, by blocking the voltage – dependent calcium channels.5 Which is the exact same mechanism of action as calcium channel blocking anti-hypertensive medications such as amlodiprine (norvasc), nicardipine (cardine SR) and verapamil (calan, verelan, covera-HS).

How to take Ginger and Contraindications:

We have already covered this in detail in chapter 4, just take a look, as there are lots of ways to take ginger...

Cardamom is a seasoning agent, which originates from India and is widely used both as a culinary agent as well as a herbal treatment. In a study of 20 patients, over a 12 week period, they noted a drop in diastolic pressure levels, from 112.59+/-1.77 down to 97.99+/-2.00, which is a drop of 8.7%.6

How to Take Cardamom:

Dosing: 3 grams of cardamom is enough to make a good impact.

Capsules: Cardamom comes in capsule form and can be taken at the rate of 1 to 3 a day depending upon dosage per capsule.

Cardamom in Food: Cardamom can easily be added to food. Here are some interesting examples:

Cardamom Sugar: Take cardamom seeds, crush them with a mortar into a powder and mix with sugar for extra taste.

Cardamom ice Cream/Whipped Cream: Crush some cardamom seeds with a mortar and then mix with ice cream/whipped cream.

1.   Take 1 tbsp. of ginger and 1/2 tsp. cardamom seeds. Mix into a container of water and milk (200ml of water and 200ml of milk).

2.   Boil the mixture until it boils once, back of and reboil, back off and reboil. Three times in total in quick succession.

3.   Filter and drink!

Cardamom Contradictions:

•   Should be avoided by pregnant ladies and breastfeeding mothers.

•   Can cause contact dermatitis, in skin sensitive individuals, via exposure to terrenes inside the seeds.

Rauvolfia serpentine

Rauvolfia serpentine is an extremely powerful and effective herb, but do take care with dosing levels and watch out for side effects. It's a great herb, but it's not for everyone!!!

Note: Because of its effectiveness Rauvolfia serpentine is mentioned here, but do take care as usually this herb is prescribed by a Homoeopathist, an Ayurvedic doctor or a Traditional Chinese Medical Practitioner. There are herbs and there are HERBS! This herb is just as powerful as any allopathic medicine and needs to be carefully monitored, so as to avoid nasty side effects, and also there are some strong contraindications to bear in mind.

Rauvolfia serpentine (snakeroot or sarpagandha in India and she gen mu in China)is a powerful and effective herb, which has been used for centuries in India and China for treating a wide variety of health conditions which includes treating insomnia, hysteria, schizophrenia, giddiness, vertigo and even snake bite. But also snakeroot is a really powerful herbal treatment, for high blood pressure.

In one study of 50 hypertensive patients, who demonstrated a minimum systolic/diastolic blood pressure level of 160/95, after 4 weeks of treatment with snakeroot, the blood pressure levels dropped on average 10 points, in both systolic and diastolic blood pressure levels. So a patient with 160/95 would show on average a drop down to 150/85!6

Snakeroot is without doubt the strongest herb mentioned in this chapter and possible in this book. It's mechanism of blood pressure reduction appears to be due to its effect on the central nervous system, which might also explain why it is so effective at treating insomnia and mental health disorders as well.7

Contraindications:

•   While snakeroot is potentially very powerful, it must also be remembered that powerful herbs often come with strong side effects, which means that it won't work for everybody. For example, in one study they noted an increase in depressive symptoms, in some patients, who were taking large doses of snakeroot.8 Snakeroot can result in a wide variety of side effects which includes depression, anxiety, nausea, convulsions, excessive sleep, vomiting and diarrhoea. So it is important to take a sufficient dose, but do not overdo it. If any

101

symptoms occur reduce the dosage and if they continue, even on a smaller dosage, then stop taking the snakeroot altogether.

• For patients with mental problems, who are on calming medications, they might find that snakeroot, when combined with their medications, may reduce their effectiveness.

• Parkinson disease patients should avoid it, as it may make their symptoms worse.

• Also pregnant ladies and breastfeeding mothers should definitely not take snakeroot!

• Do not use heavy machinery after imbibing snakeroot, as it might result in feelings of sleepiness.

• Do not take if you are suffering from gastric problems.

• It clashes with alcohol. Do not take at the same time as consuming alcohol.

In summary snakeroot is a really powerful herb, but dosing has to be maintained at a low level. Also, just like ginseng (another potent Chinese medicinal herb) it might make sense to cycle of off snakeroot, every now and again, so as to protect the body from overuse of this herb. Possibly two months on and one month off, might be a conservative approach to taking this powerful herb!

Dosage:

Snakeroot comes either in dry root form or in a capsule or as a powder, or as a tincture. In capsule or powder form, take 2grams a day divided into two servings. As a tincture, take 12 drops, 3 times daily.

Also, another more powerful way is to take desiccated (dry) snakeroot and mix it with water. Take one piece of root and leave it overnight in 7 ounces (100ml's) of water, strain and serve. Then put the same root back into another 7 ounces of water, and again imbibe before going to bed. If a small quantity of root is used, it is enough for two servings, if a bigger piece of root is used, it will be enough for 4 servings (2 days' supply). It's easy to know, simply check the taste out, if it is extremely bitter then keep reusing the root up to a total of 2 days, and 4 servings.

In this raw form, rauvolfia serpentine is very powerful and very effective. The only downside been that it is difficult to know exactly how many grams are been taken. So if you take this route, it is an intuitive choice, so see how you feel on it and adjust accordingly.

Cinnamon/Cardamom/Ginger

We have covered each of these herbs earlier (cinnamon for cold and flu and diabetic symptoms/ cardamom for high blood pressure/ginger for cold and flu, nausea and high blood pressure). The good thing is that all three works really well, at treating diabetic symptoms. In a study comparing cinnamon, cardamom and ginger, they note that each one had a noticeable effect on blood sugar levels, and that in particular cinnamon had the greatest effect in lowering blood sugar levels.[1]

In another study, on the effects of cinnamon, they took 79 patients and split them into a placebo group and cinnamon group. The cinnamon group were put on 3 grams of cinnamon a day and after 4 months the cinnamon group demonstrated a 10.3% reduction in blood sugar levels! [2]

How to take Cinnamon, Garlic and Cardamom:

Any of the ways outlined earlier will be effective at treating diabetes.

Aloe Vera

We have already touched on the role of aloe Vera, in helping stomach problems, well aloe Vera is also helpful in treating diabetes. Aloe Vera reduces blood lipids (fats) in the blood, which is an issue for diabetic patiens.[3] In another study, on

104

the effectiveness of aloe Vera, they noted a significant reduction in blood glucose levels, within two weeks and triglycerides within 4 weeks.4 Furthermore, it helps to decrease swelling and brings about quicker healing of wound injuries 5, which of course is useful as diabetics have to be careful that they do not develop necrotic tissue.

How to take Aloe Vera for Diabetes:

Two tbsp. of aloe Vera juice per day will make a noticeable improvement.

Bilberry Extract

Bilberries (vaccinium myrtillus) are berries, and like most berries that possess many health benefits which include strengthening blood vessels, improvement of circulation, it prevents cell damage, possibly it might help with retinopathy and also it is good for reducing blood sugar levels.

In particular bilberries contain anthocyanosides, which promote blood vessel strength and which may protect diabetic patients from developing retinal damage 6. Prevention is always better than cure, and diabetics must remember that diabetes isn't simply about high blood sugar, that the high blood sugar levels are damaging to the body and that not only must the blood sugar be lowered but also it is necessary to protect against the side effects.

The side effects of diabetes, in general tend to be heart damage (as a consequence of high triglyceride levels), kidney damage (as a result of cardiovascular damage), nerve damage (which can lead to necrosis), necrosis (which can lead to amputation) and retinopathy. So this quality of bilberries, is really important.

Bilberry may have some effect also in lowering blood sugar, but the main benefit of bilberries is as a possible defence against retinopathy.

Since retinopathy is a fairly common occurrence with diabetics, who have diabetes over a period of many years, it makes sense to take bilberries as a possible preventative measure, and also bilberries are really tasty, so it's all win win!

The other important side effect, of bilberries, is on blood circulation and vascular health, with research suggesting that bilberries possess vascular protective qualities.7 Lack of good blood circulation and arterial damage, in diabetics, result in a crescendo of negative side effects. Bilberries will help to protect the cardiovascular system, which is really helpful!

How to take Bilberries for Diabetes:

Approximately 20 to 60grams a day produce a good result, and up to 160mg of bilberry extract have been taken by people who have retinopathy with some promising results.8

Bilberry extract can be found in capsules or powder. Take capsules as per grams suggested, of bilberry recommended per day. As a powder it, can be mixed with food or drinks. Also, bilberries can be acquired as crushed bilberries, which once again can be mixed with foods. This is ideal for making shakes, or even for mixing with ice cream or whipped cream to make a really tasty and healthy snack!

Bilberry Tea:

If you can get your hands on bilberry leaves, it is possible to make a delicious bilberry tea.

1.   Boil water and add in 1 gram, which are 2 the spoonful's of chopped dried bilberry leaves.

2.   Leave too steep for 10 minutes.

3.   Filter and serve.

Bilberry Contraindications:

•   Bilberry may make diabetic medicine over effective, consequently diabetics need to check their sugar levels regular, when they start to take bilberry, and adjust the level of medications which they take accordingly.

•   Medications which slow blood clotting (anticoagulant / antiplatelet drugs) are made more effective by bilberry intake. Since bilberries already slow down blood clotting, the combination of bilberries with blood clotting medication may result in excessive bleeding and bruising. Examples of these drugs include clopidogrel (Plavix), ibuprofen (Advil, Motrin, others) and warfarin.

Fenugreek

Fenugreek is an annual plant, in the family Fabaceae, and is widely used as a food ingredient in Asian foods, such as curries and other Indian recipes.

Fenugreek also possess a wide variety of health benefits, which includes the ability of reduce cholesterol, protect the heart, relives constipation, benefits the kidneys and also helps to relieve diabetic symptoms.

Fenugreek seed (trigonella foenum graecum) are high in soluble fibre, which aids blood sugar control as it slows down the absorption of carbohydrates.

In a study on fenugreek, they took 25 patients, splitting them into two groups, a placebo group and a fenugreek group. They gave the fenugreek group 1gram a day of fenugreek, and after two months the fenugreek group saw a noticeable reduction in blood sugar levels, as well as an improvement in insulin senility and a decrease in unhealthy cholesterol levels.9

How to take Fenugreek:

On scientific experiments, fenugreek has been taken anywhere from 2 grams to 100 grams per day. So this is quite a variance. The best advice is to take a smallish dosage of fenugreek, once and twice a day, and see how it goes and adjust if necessary.

Fenugreek seeds are readily available in stores as a culinary food extract. It can come as seeds and as powders and pastes.

Roasted Fenugreek: Fenugreek seeds can be
roasted and added into curries.

Fenugreek Powders and Pastes: Fenugreek can be added into food as a powder or as a paste.

Fenugreek tea:

1.   Boil water.

2.   Add in 2tbsp of fenugreek leaves.

3.   Leave to simmer for 10 minutes.

4.   Strain and serve.

Fenugreek Contraindications:

•   Fenugreek seeds may make diabetic medications more effective, consequently diabetics should keep an eye on their medications and reduce as need be so as to avoid low blood sugar levels.

•   Medications which slow blood clotting (anticoagulant / antiplatelet drugs) are made more effective by fenugreek intake. Since febugreek already slow down blood clotting, the combination of fenugreek with blood clotting medication may result in excessive bleeding and bruising. Examples of these drugs include clopidogrel (plavix), ibuprofen (advil, motrin, others) and warfarin.

Evening Primrose Oil is a great supplement , which works well on menopausal symptoms, osteoporosis care, skincare, anti-inflammatory properties and it's good for cardiovascular health, and of course nerve health!

Evening Primrose Oil contains gamma linoleic acid, which helps in repairing damaged nerve cells. In clinical trials, when they gave 480mg of Evening Primrose Oil, for a period of one year, the participants demonstrated signs of nerve repair10.

This is very helpful for diabetics, as many diabetics suffer nerve damage, especially to the feet and end up getting cuts, which become gangrenous and then this leads onto sever problems, which can end up with amputation of the lower limbs!

So definitely Evening Primrose Oil is a must for any diabetic patient who wants to prevent nerve damage!

Black Cohosh

Black Cohosh (Actaea racemosa, Cimicifuga racemosa) is a flowering plant of the family Ranunculaceae. Black cohosh is a popular herb, for women suffering menopausal symptoms, but it does appear to have a mixed effect on those who take it.

In a study, comparing black cohosh to oestrogen replacement therapy, they found that 40mg of black cohosh per day to be equivalent in effectiveness to 0.6mg of oestrogen replacements. In this study it was particularly noted, that black cohosh was just as effective at improving bone density and helping to relieve vaginal dryness as its oestrogen replacement equaivalent.[1] However in other studies, black cohosh has demonstrated considerably less effectiveness, than actual hormone replacement therapy (HRT).[2]

For example, in one study[2] they noted a statistically notable difference between HRT and black cohosh. Looking at various studies, the results for black cohosh appear to be very mixed. Black Cohosh is mentioned in this chapter, because it is a popular herb for treating menopausal symptoms, but it must be borne in mind that it appears to work for some and not for others.

It's worth trying out black cohosh and seeing if it helps to relieve symptoms, in some cases it may, but it probably acts as a supplement to HRT rather than as a replacement.

How to take Black Cohosh:

Black cohosh is usually taking in capsule form and can be taken in anywhere from 8mg to 160mg per day.

Black Cohosh Contraindications:

•   Atorvastatin (Lipitor) mixed with black cohosh may increase the likelihood of liver damage.

•   Cisplatin (Platinol-AQ) might lose some of its effectiveness when combined with black cohosh.

•   Medications changed by the liver, cytochrome P450 2D6 and CYP2D6 substrates, may take longer to absorb and may have more side effects if combined with black cohosh.

•   Some medications can harm the liver (these are known as Hepatotoxic drugs) mixed with black cohosh may increase the likelihood of liver damage.

Soy

Soya is an extremely popular food, and is used equally as a food source as well as a food supplement, for example, soya is very popular as a protein supplement. Also soya is noted for its oestrogen boosting abilities. So much so, that men are warned from taking too much soya lest they end up with an imbalance between their testosterone and oestrogen levels, resulting in such unpleasant side effects as "man boobs" (male fatty breast tissue enlargement) and low testosterone levels. Needless to say, this same ability to boost oestrogen, while not good in the case of men, is very good in the case of women!

In a study of 80 women, they placed half of them on 100mg a day of soya, for a period of 4 months, saw a decrease in menopausal symptoms and also a decline in cholesterol levels.3

So far so good, however, in another study carried out on 69 participants, over 24 weeks found no significant improvement in menopausal symptoms!4

What are we to think?

Well soya does promote oestrogen production, and certainly in some cases it works well, but maybe it's effectiveness depends upon the present level of oestrogen production in the ladies been tested.

So like black cohosh, the best advice is to try it out and see how well it works.

How to take Soy:

There are an endless number of ways of imbibing soya, all of which will result in the ingestion of an adequate soy supplementation. Examples including boiled soybeans, tempeh, soya milk, tofu, tofu yoghurt, soya cheese and of course soya protein powders.

Soya Contraindications:

•   Soya combined with Monoamine Oxidase Inhibitors (MAOI's) can result in elevated blood pressure levels, if the person consumes a charge quantity of fermented soya, combined with MAOI's.

•   Antibiotics may be less effective when mixed with soy products.

•   Tamoxifen (Nolvadex), a drug used to treat oestrogen-sensitive cancers, may be made less effective when combined with soya.

•   Warfarin, a drug used to slow blood clotting, may be made less effective when combined with soya.

Ginseng

Gingseng is a perennial plant with fleshy roots, belonging to the genus panax of the araliaceae family. Gingseng is famous for its sexual enhancing properties; however gingseng possesses many benefits which includes anti-inflammatory properties, memory enhancement, cancer prevention, erectile dysfunction, libido boosting, immunity boosting and the prevention and treatment of cold's and flu's.

Ginseng is a famous herb, used in traditional Chinese Medicine (TCM), and it is notable that from a TCM point of view ginseng boosts yang energy (active energy), and since menopause represents a drop in active energy, it makes sense that ginseng may well improve some of the symptoms.

Interestingly, in a study on the effects of ginseng on both menopausal symptoms and cardiovascular health, of ladies in menopause, noted that a significant improvement in the symptoms of menopause, a drop in cholesterol levels and a

114

noticeable reduction in carotid intima-media thickness, which is an indicator of cardiovascular health.5

From a TCM point of view, menopause is simply a rapid drop off in yang energy (active energy), which results in symptoms because of its suddenness!

Also, they noted in this study, that blood serum oestrogen levels remained low, so ginseng (RG – red ginseng was the particular ginseng used in this study) isn't attempting to be a hormone replacement, rather it's a symptom improver. From a TCM point of view, this makes sense because in TCM menopause is simply a rapid drop off in yang energy (active energy), which results in symptoms because of its suddenness.

A herb like ginseng, boosts the yang energy thus reducing symptoms, so really it can be seen as a way of boosting and supporting this transition in a ladies life, after all menopause is not an illness rather it is a natural part of life!

How to take Ginseng

Dosing is usually anywhere from 100mg to 400mg's per day.

Ginseng Capsules: Can be easily taken put several capsules a day.

Ginseng Extract: Ginseng can be taken in tincture form. Just add 10 - 30 drops of extract to any beverage and drink.

Ginseng Tea

If you can get some ginseng extract, it is possible to make a refreshing cup of ginseng tea.

1.   Boil 150ml of water

2.   Add in several slices of ginseng

3.   Leave to simmer for 2 hours.

4.   Strain and serve.

An Important Warning on Ginseng Usage

Ginseng is a great herb, but it is a lot like caffeine in that too much can be bad for you. In particular people, who are anxious and depressed, should be careful about its usage. It may help some anxious and depressed people while making other people, who suffer from these symptoms, far worse.

Another thing, is that ginseng is too strong took use all year round, you have to take a break. After 2 to 3 months usage, stop for a month, it will help in the long run.

From a TCM point of view, too much yang (active energy) will actually result in too little young (nurturing energy), which results in feeling burnt out and emotional. In the orient ginseng is widely used by middle aged men for erectile dysfunction and as a libido booster. However, many of them end up developing anxiety and depression, as a result!

So don't under estimate ginseng because it's just a herb, well it's a powerful herb. Also, a lot of advertising is misleading, as supplement companies want your

116

money and do not care about your health. Ginseng is great, but use it carefully and wisely!

Ginger Contraindications:

•   Ginseng is a very powerful yang herb. It is terrific at boosting the system but, while a good way to treat physical exhaustion it impacts negatively on people who are suffering mental emotional burnout, as these people are suffering from ying defiance (nurturing energy) and the increase in yang will actual aggravate the nervous emotional side effects.

•   Ginseng is taken with excessive amounts of caffeine might be hazardous to the nervous system.

•   Ginseng may reduce blood sugar levels, so diabetic should monitor their sugar levels while on ginseng.

•   Monoamine Oxidise Inhibitor (MAOI's) may interact baldy with ginseng, (anticoagulant / antiplatelet drugs) may become less effective at slowing down blood clotting if combined with ginseng.

A Note on Treating Menopause via Herbal Remedies

In this chapter we mentioned black cohosh, soya and ginseng. Ginseng has a pretty good reputation, for treating symptoms of menopause, while black cohosh and soy have demonstrate mixed results. Also, other popular herbs such as Kava, St John's Worth and Evening Primrose all have mixed reports. Why is this so?

The Effect of Complimentary Therapies as a Means of Slowing Down and Balancing the Hormonal Drop of Experienced during Menopause

According to TCM, the symptoms of menopause are a natural stage in a woman's life and they arise because of a sudden drop of in yang energy (active energy).However, TCM also tells us that the symptoms can be reduced by boosting yang energy. Now one way to boost yang energy, is to take HRT (hormone replacement therapy), but other approaches include herbs, yoga, acupuncture, homeopathy and other complimentary medicines (which boost the yang energy and hep the natural drop off in hormonal levels to have a far more gently down curve), also have role to play.

Take a look at the diagram above, in this diagram we can see that normal oestrogen levels and HRT oestrogen levels are both listed as been 100. This isn't meant to be a literal interpretation as to oestrogen levels, but rather it represents normal levels, so HRT allows hormone levels to be normal. When we look at menopausal symptoms we see over a period of time, of approximately 10 years an enormous drop off in female hormone levels.

Finally we see a line entitled as complementary therapies, which again is not to be taken literally, but rather it represents the effects of complimentary therapies on female hormone levels. So when complimentary therapies, such as herbs, yoga, aryuveda, homeopathy, acupuncture, tai chi, chi gong etc. along with regular exercise and a healthy diet, the drop off in hormone levels is more gradual. Inevitably the hormonal levels still drop off considerably over a 10 year period, however, the drop as we can see in the diagram is gradual rather than sudden.

The result of this gradual drop off is a reduction, and even in some cases, an eradication of some menopausal symptoms. It is this sudden drop of in hormone levels, and subtle energy levels in the female body, which produce most of the symptoms in the first place. Taking a complimentary approach will definitely make the menopause a far more comfortable transition.

But surely there is no comparison between HRT and complementary medicine?

Well this is true, after all complimentary medicine cannot be equivalent to bio-identical hormones!

What we must remember, when treating menopause, is that herbs cannot compete with HRT. Hormone replacement therapy is really powerful. If we take a look at steroids, in sports for example, steroids are hormones, in particular they are, male hormones (testosterone) and derivatives and they boost endurance, strength, size and pretty much all performance parameters, simply because of the boosting effect of adding a hormone.

In the case of hormone replacement therapy (both male and female), those hormones (oestrogen in women and testosterone in men) makes a huge improvement. Herbs are good but they are not that good!

Even in herbs which boost oestrogen, they will only make a small difference, and this might be why scientific results of herbs demonstrate such mixed results, because the oestrogen levels of different ladies undergoing menopause will vary. Furthermore one lady could have lower oestrogen levels, than another lady, and yet have fewer symptoms. Why? Because of genetics. So there are so many variables both in oestrogen levels and symptoms, so keep this in mind.

It is unlikely that any herb can replace hormone replacement therapy. But this is not a bad thing, for example diabetic women are usually advised to avoid HRT, because of a negative impact of increased oestrogen levels on diabetics. Well in herbs which only boost oestrogen to a small degree, maybe this will provide them a boost.

If you are undergoing the symptoms of menopause and either want to avoid using HRT or want to take herbs as well as HRT, in an effort to reduce or eradicate symptoms, then by all means try out these herbs. But do realise that results vary, and take an experimental approach to herbal intake. Try out a low dosage and observe, over a few weeks, and then increase the dosage and see again for a few weeks. If the result is good keep going, if the results are lacking try another herb.

It is better to try out one herb, at a time, so as to see which is working well for you. Also, herbs are slow to act, so give it a few weeks to be fair. Unlike HRT which hits very quickly, herbs are slow to act, but this doesn't mean that they are no good, rather it simply means that they are slow to work.

Good News from Traditional Chinese Medicine

Finally, remember that if one herb or complimentary medicine or even if HRT, fail to work well for you, then experiment with other options. For one thing is for sure, menopause does not have to be terribly incapacitating. Understand that your symptoms, are a result of a sudden drop off in hormone levels, as well as a sudden drop off in subtle energies within the body, and that definitely the symptoms of menopause can be reduced to a considerable degree. But nobody is going to hand it to you on a plate. Every person has a unique body and a unique approach is required, in order to make sure that relieve is achieved. Don't give up, take heart and you will get there through a little bit of trial and error!

Thank You

I hope you have enjoyed this book and found it interesting. These herbs are very powerful and are a simple way to support you through the recovery process. But do remember they are a support so don't simply swap allopathic medications for herbs. Both allopathic and herbal formulations are simply there to asset you while you recover.

If you like this book please leave a review for it and for more interesting and helpful information, on every suspect of physical, mental, emotional and spiritual health, please visit my website:

www.healbodymindandpspirit.com

Thanks once again for taking the time out to read this book.

Dermot Farrell

Free Gifts

Bonus #1 – Grab Free Books!!!!!!!!

As a way of saying thank you for downloading this book I would like to give you two free books, which are available exclusively for my readers. The free book "Juicing for Health – 35 Juicing Recipes for Everyday Health Problems", is packed full of useful healthy juice recipes and Success Hacks - 31 Mind-Set Hacks to Increase Productivity and Career Success, is packed full of helpful mind hacks for developing a more dynamic and enjoyable lifestyle!

Please go to my blog page and sign up here:

www.healbodymindandspirit.com

You will receive the two free eBooks, plus weekly updates and even free eBooks!

Bonus#2 - Bonus Video Series

You can check out my YouTube channel, which has lots of health related videos

Please copy the following link into your browser, to access an introduction to herbal remedies video. If you then go to my channel and click playlists, you will find lots of videos on herbs for health:

http://y2u.be/rWpgVltW4dw

If you find it too awkward to type in this code, then you can also find my channel by typing in **www.healbodymindandspirit.com** into the YouTube search bar!

About the Author

Dermot Farrell was born and raised in Ireland. He first took an interest in mental health back in the 1990's when he studied psychoanalytic studies, hypnotherapy and clinical psychoanalytical psychotherapy. While he learned a great deal about the workings of the mind, at this time, his interest in healing encouraged him to attend classes in Traditional Chinese Medicine and Acupuncture, finally culminating in him receiving a clinical diploma in 2005.

Since then Dermot has ran a TCM (Traditional Chinese Medical) clinic for a considerable period of time and also he has taken to writing about a variety of topics. His most recent writings are found on his blog www.healbodymindandspirit.com

Dermot has learned, from his experience, the importance of balance in the three key domains of our life, which are physical, mental-emotional and spiritual wellbeing. His approach to healing is infinitely practical and is based upon the need to balance each of these aspects of our life, in order to regain a balanced state.

Furthermore, he is interested in moving the western/eastern medical discourse forward. Believing in the virtue of both western (allopathic) and eastern (complimentary) healing systems and is continually pushing for an integrated approach to healing. As the old saying goes "doctors differ, patients die!" demonstrates the need for everyone, who is interested in health and healing, to work together towards learning more about the causes of ill-health and the techniques of rebalancing health and reaching out in a humanistic way to help our patients, regain their health.

As well as his interest in healing Dermot possesses an interest in spirituality too. In 1999 Dermot began to meditate in an Indian system of Raja Yoga, known as Sahaj Marg. With an ardent interest in spirituality as well as physical, mental and emotional healing, Dermot presently resides in India with his wife and son.

Dermot can be contacted at admin@healbodymindandspirit.com

Website: www.healbodymindandspirit.com

APPENDIX ONE

Herbal Remedies – Popular Herbal Teas, Tinctures and Recipes

Chapter One – Anxiety

Kava Kava Tea

1.   Take 3tbsp's of kava kava in with 3 cups of water.

2.   Heat for 5 minutes.

3.   Strain and pour.

Also, Kava Kava can be mixed with sprite or 7up or even coconut milk!

Passionflower Tea

1.   Grind 2 grams of passionflower (per cup) into a fine powder.

2.   Add the ground leaves into a cup of water and bring to the boil.

3.   Leave to simmer for 20 minutes.

4.   Strain and drink.

Passionflower Tincture

1.   To make a tincture, we have to mix the plant material with a liquid which will suck out the chemical compounds from the herb, this liquid is called the menstruum. The ratio necessary with is 2:1. The menstruum is usually alcohol, but apple cider vinegar can be used instead. The menstruum also also helps to preserve the tincture, so the tincture can be used over a long period of time. Brandy, vodka, and grain alcohol are used as the alcohol base, do not use beer! It's necessary for the menstruum to be high in alcohol, so as to preserve the tincture.

2.   To make the menstruum, mix in alcohol/apple cider vinegar to a ratio of 3:1 with water and the menstruum with the passionflower with a ratio of 2:1.

3.   Take 3 ounces (90grams) of alcohol/vinegar to a ratio of about 1 ounce (30 grams) of water. Then place the mix into a blender and blend. The flower now has to be chopped and ground. Then add in 2 ounces (60grams) of passionflower with 4 ounces (120 grams) of menstruum.

4.   Then pour into a glass container (do not use plastic), and leave it in a dark cool place.

5.   Shake every day for the next 14 days.

6.   Strain through several layers of cheesecloth and squeeze out the essence.

7.   Leave the mix which remains to settle for 12 to 16 hours, then pour out the clear liquid from the top of the jar, which is called the decant.

8.   The decant can now be Stored in a dark glass container in a dark place which should also be cold.

When you want to take it just take out a tincture dropper and use one to two drops anywhere, three to five times daily.

This tincture will last a long time because of the preserving qualities of alcohol/vinegar.

Chamomile Tea

1.   Boil water.

2.   Add one teaspoon of dried chamomile leaves.

3.   Simmer for twenty minutes.

4.   Strain and serve.

Chapter Four – Allergies

Stinging Nettle Tea

1.   Add 1ounze (16grams) of stinging netle powder.

2.   Boil water

3.   Add stinging nettles to the water and leave to simmer for 20 minutes.

4.   Strain and serve.

Stinging Nettle Infusion

1.   Half fill a pint sized jar with dried nettles.

2.   Add boiling water. Secure the lid, using some wax paper so as to seal in the vapour.

3.   Let the jar sit for at least 4 hours.

4. Filter and place the infusions in a glass jar and keep in the refrigerator.

The stinging nettles infusion can be heated up and drank just like a tea, the only difference been that the infusion is much stronger than the herbal tea. Experiment with each and see how it feels for you.

Stinging nettle tea and infusions will keep for 3 to 4 days.

Chapter Four – Cold and Flu

Thyme Tea

1. Add 2 tbsps. of fresh thyme to 1 cup if boiling water.

2. Steam for 10 minutes.

3. Filter and serve.

Exotic Thyme Tea

1. Add 2 tbsps. of fresh thyme to 1 cup if boiling water.

2. Steam for 10 minutes.

3. Add 1 tbsp. of honey, 1 tsp. of turmeric, 1 tops of cayenne paper and 1 tsp. of grated ginger.

4. Add 1 tbsp. of lemon juice.

5. Filter and serve.

1.   To make a tincture, we have to mix the plant material with a liquid which will suck out the chemical compounds from the herb, this liquid is called the menstruum. The ratio necessary with is 2:1. The menstruum is usually alcohol, but apple cider vinegar can be used instead. The menstruum also also helps to preserve the tincture, so the tincture can be used over a long period of time. Brandy, vodka, and grain alcohol are used as the alcohol base, do not use beer! It's necessary for the menstruum to be high in alcohol, so as to preserve the tincture.

2.   To make the menstruum, mix in alcohol/apple cider vinegar to a ratio of 3:1 with water and the menstruum with the thyme with a ratio of 2:1.

3.   Take 3 ounces (90grams) of alcohol/vinegar to a ratio of about 1 ounce (30 grams) of water. Then place the mix into a blender and blend. The flower now has to be chopped and ground. Then add in 2 ounces (60grams) of thyme with 4 ounces (120 grams) of menstruum.

4.   Then pour into a glass container (do not use plastic), and leave it in a dark cool place.

5.   Shake every day for the next 14 days.

6.   Strain through several layers of cheesecloth and squeeze out the essence.

7.   Leave the mix which remains to settle for 12 to 16 hours, then pour out the clear liquid from the top of the jar, which is called the decant.

8.   The decant can now be Stored in a dark glass container in a dark place which should also be cold.

When you want to take it just take out a tincture dropper and use one to two drops anywhere, three to five times daily.

This tincture will last a long time because of the preserving qualities of alcohol/vinegar.

1.   Add 2 cups of dried elderberries to 4 glasses of water and add 1 cinnamon stick, and/or 1 teaspoon of garlic powder.

2.   Boil the mixture and then simmer for 5 minutes, or until the mixture has been reduced by half its volume.

3.   Remove from the stove, mix the berry solution with a large spoon or ladle, then strain the mixture.

4.   This syrup can be used as is, or if you want to add flavour then add in some honey, gently heating the syrup/honey mixture for a couple of minutes(but not boiling), then take the mixture and pour it into a glass bottle.

Chapter Five – Headaches

Feverfew Tea

1.   Pour one cup of boiling water over one tablespoon full of dried feverfew leaves.

2.   Steep for thirty to sixty minutes.

3.   Strain and serve

Stream Inhalation: Here you add several drops of Eucalyptus oil to a large bowl of boiled water, place a towel over your head and breathe in deeply. This is one of the most satisfying ways to take this oil as relief is instantaneous and deeply satisfying.

Dilution and Application: This is a little more direct than steam inhalation, it can be effective, and the good thing is that it is less cumbersome than steam inhalation, but some people find it irritating, so try it out and see how it works for you.

Add a few drop of Eucalyptus oil in with non-irritating oil, and then rub it directly onto the facial area. In diluted form Eucalyptus can be really potent with little or no irritation.

Direct Application: Is for people who have very insensitive skin. This is really easy; simply rub the oil into the sensitive area, that's it.

Chapter Six – Stomach

Lemon Juice

A tasty way to take lemon juice is as follows:

- Add one teaspoon of lemon juice to a 200ml glass of water.

- Add a teaspoon of honey

- Mix well and drink

For something a little more exotic try:

1.   Take a 200ml glass of water and add one teaspoon of lemon juice.

2.   Add a teaspoon of honey, one teaspoon of ginger juice and a pinch of black pepper.

3.   Mix well and drink.

Chapter 7 – Nausea

Peppermint

Peppermint Tea: Peppermint tea is the most famous, and tasty way, to take Peppermint. Peppermint tea is widely available at health food shops and even supermarkets. You can also make your own Peppermint tea, as follows:

1.   Boil water.

2.   Place peppermint leaves or extract in a cup of tea pot and pour water.

3.   Leave to soak for about five minutes.

4.   Filter and drink.

1.   Wash the peppermint leaves and chop them.

2.   Place them in a jar with carrier oil, such as olive oil, for instance. Seal the jar, ideally with wax paper on the lid and leave to soak for 24 hours.

3.   Strain the oil and add additional peppermint leaves and olive oil reseal and leave for another 24 hours.

4.   Repeat every day for 5 days.

5.   Finally remove the peppermint leaves and strain the oil into a glass container.

Cloves

Clove Tea: Simply boil 250ml of water and add 1 tsp of clove powder (or 4 clove pods) to it, filter and drink.

Cloves and Honey: Add a small amount of ground and roasted clove pods to 1stp of honey, mix and drink up to 4 times a day.

Clove Oil Inhalation: Simply sprinkle a few drops of clove oil onto your pillow at night, or on your handkerchief during the day. This is ideal for pregnant ladies suffering from morning sickness and busy people who are worried about making a scene in public.

Cumin Tea: Boil 250ml of water and then add the cloves, and leave to steep for ten minutes. Filter out the cumin seeds and drink.

Fennel Tea: Fennel tea is a popular item in most health food stores. But it can also be easily be made at home by boiling water, mixing in some fennel seeds and stepping for 10 minutes, then filtering and drinking.

How to take Baking Soda:

Baking Soda mixed with Cleanser: When trying out baking soda, for the first time, this is a good idea, as it is a way for you to assess its effectiveness and make sure that you do not have a bad reaction to it.

1.   Simply add half a teaspoon of baking soda to your cleanser, mix it and then message into the skin.

2.   Wash off.

3.   Immediately rub in moisturiser

Face Mask: Face masks are a great way to reduce inflammation and redness of the skin.

1.   Cleanse the face with a gentle cleanser.

2.   Mix 2 teaspoons of baking soda with water and make a paste.

3.   Apply to the skin and leave it for 15 minutes. If it stings a little then ok, if it is too irritating then take it off. Also, do try the cleanser approach first, so to assess for any allergic reactions. Also, the first time you put on the baking soda mask, just try it for a few minutes, wash it off and check for any reactions, always be careful when applying anything to your skin for the first time.

4.   Wash off and apply moisturiser.

Cleansing Spots: Because baking soda is such a good anti-inflammatory, it is very good at spot reduction. Also this particular approach is very useful for anyone who has very sensitive skin, whereby the cleanser and mask approach is possible to irritating.

1.   Mix a little bit of baking soda and water and apply directly to a pimple, cyst or inflamed area.

2.   Leave on for 20 minutes.

3.   Let it harden.

4.   Then remove and apply some moisturiser.

Apple Cider Vinegar

Note: Never apply undiluted to the skin and Apple Cider Vinegar is a strong base!

Apple Cider Vinegar Toner: Mix Apple Cider Vinegar to water at the ratio of 50:50

More Exotic Toner: Mix Apple Cider Vinegar with green tea or aloe Vera gel or witch hazel.

Direct Application: Mix ACV with water and soak a cotton bud. Then rub on the skin in affected areas.

How to use Tea Tree Oil:

Cleanser and Moisturizer: Simply add a few drops of tea tree oil in with your cleanser or moisturiser.

Facial Scrub:

1.   Mix half a cup of sugar with 1 tbsp. of honey, ¼ coup of sesame or olive oil with 10 drops of tea tree oil in a small bowl.

2.   Gently scrub the face for 5 minutes.

3.   Rinse off with Luke warm water and dry.

Facial masks:

Here are three variations:

1.   Take 2 tbsp. of green clay powder and mix in 3 to 4 drops of tea tree oil. Add water and mix so as to form a paste. Apply onto the face and leave it for 20 minutes. Rinse with lukewarm water and dry.

2.   Mix 1 tsp. of jojoba oil with 3 drops of tea tree oil and add in a finely chopped tomato. Mix into a puree and apply on as a face mask. Leave for 20 minutes then use some arm water to wash it off.

3.   Take ¼ cup of plain yoghurt and add in 5 drop soft tea tree oil. Apply directly to the face and leave for 20 minutes. Wash off with lukewarm water and dry.

Spot Treatment:

1.   Take a few drops of aloe vera gel and add in a couple of drops of oil into it. If you don't have aloe vera simply use honey in its place.

2.   Apply mixture directly to pimple, or area of sensitive skin.

Apply to Pimples Directly:

1.   Add a couple of drop soft tea tree oil to a cotton bud.

2.   Dab the affected area with the cotton bud.

Chapter 10 – High Blood Pressure

Cinnamon Tea

Cinnamon can also be taken as a tea.

1.   Add water to a stick of Ceylon cinnamon.

2.   Boil slowly so as to release the cinnamon from the stick.

3.   Eventually the water should turn a mild brown colour; this should take about 15 minutes.

Leave it to sit for 15 to 20 minutes, so as to settle down. You will know it is ready when the colour suddenly changes from brown to a red colour.

Cardamom

Cardamom Sugar: Take cardamom seeds, crush them with a mortar into a powder and mix with sugar for extra taste.

Cardamom ice Cream/Whipped Cream: Crush some cardamom seeds with a mortar and then mix with ice cream/whipped cream.

Cardamom and Ginger Tea:

1. Take 1 tbsp. of ginger and 1/2 tsp cardamom seeds. Mix into a container of water and milk (200ml of water and 200ml of milk).

2. Boil the mixture until it boils once, back of and recoil, back off and recoil. Three times in total in quick succession.

3. Filter and drink!

Bilberry Tea

If you can get your hands on bilberry leaves, it is possible to make a delicious bilberry tea.

1. Boil water and add in 1 gram, which are 2 the spoonful's of chopped dried bilberry leaves.

2. Leave too steep for 10 minutes.

3. Filter and serve.

Fenugreek

Roasted Fenugreek: Fenugreek seeds can be roasted and added into curries.

Fenugreek Powders and Pastes: Fenugreek can be added into food as a powder or as a paste.

1.   Boil water.

2.   Add in 2tbsp of fenugreek leaves.

3.   Leave to simmer for 10 minutes.

4.   Strain and serve.

Chapter 12 – Menopause

Gingseng

Ginseng Extract: Ginseng can be taken in tincture form. Just add 10 - 30 drops of extract to any beverage and drink.

Ginseng tea

If you can get some ginseng extract, it is possible to make a refreshing cup of ginseng tea.

1.   Boil 150ml of water

2.   Add in several slices of ginseng

3.   Leave to simmer for 2 hours.

4.   Strain and serve.

Appendix 2

Kava Kava	<ul><li>Anti-anxietic</li><li>stomach upset</li><li>Lessens fatigue</li><li>Infection treatment</li><li>Arthritis and rheumatism</li><li>Asthma</li><li>Urinary disorders</li><li>Relaxant</li><li>Headaches</li><li>Cramps and muscle pain</li><li>Insomnia</li><li>Prevent infection</li><li>General tonic</li><li>Mild sedative and tranquilizer</li></ul>
St John's Wort	<ul><li>Anti-depressive</li><li>Anxiety</li><li>SAD (Seasonal affective disorder)</li><li>PMS(Premenstrual syndrome)</li><li>Insomnia</li><li>Wounds</li><li>Burns</li><li>Haemorrhoids</li></ul>
Valerian	<ul><li>Valerian eases menstrual cramps.</li><li>Helps to relieve insomnia</li><li>It eases stomach cramps</li><li>Eases mental tension</li></ul>
Passionflower	<ul><li>Insomnia</li></ul>

	• Anxiety • Pain relief • Anti – depressant • Menstrual issues • High blood pressure • Drug withdrawal
Chamomile	• Anxiety • Anti-depressive • Relieves nausea • Irritable Bowel Syndrome (IBS) • Good for stomach ulcers • Anti-allergic • Headache relief • Skin irritations
Butterbur	• Preventing migraine headaches • Asthma • Hay fever • Mental relief for people who are undergoing physical pain
Quercetin	• Respiratory system • Cardiovascular health • High blood pressure • Anti-stress
Stinging Nettle	• Anti-allergic • Urinary tract infections • Skin health • Digestive health
Thyme	• Stops coughing • Respiratory inflammation • Lowers blood pressure • Boosts immunity
Elderberry	• Boosts the immune system

	• Reduces symptoms of cold and flu • Reduces sinusitis • Aids weight loss
Garlic	• Fights colds and flu's • Reduces blood pressure • Reduces cholesterol levels • Fights dementia • Improves bone health
Honey	• **Anti-bacterial, anti-fungal** • **Reduces cough and respiratory irritation** • **Regulates blood sugar levels** • **Good for burns** • **Good for cuts**
Kudzu	• Cluster Headaches • Anti-cancerous • Softens menopausal symptoms
Eucalyptus	• Sinus headaches • Mental exhaustion • Respiratory difficulties • Muscle pain • Dental problems • Skin care • Diabetes • Lice • **Pneumonia** • **Mouth wash**
Apple cider vinegar	• Stomach • Antibacterial/antimicrobial • Good for blood sugar regulation • Weight Loss • Heart health • Anti-cancerous properties

Lemon Juice	• Good for sore throats • Weight loss • Kidney stones • Digestion • Balances pH levels • Reduces fevers
Aloe Vera Juice	• Digestion • Constipation • Regulates blood sugar levels • Colon cleaning • Detoxifies the body • Improves circulation • Regulates blood pressure • Strengthens the immune system • Anti-cancerous properties • Anti-inflammatory
Ginger	• Nausea • Muscle pain and soreness • Anti-inflammatory • Lowers blood sugar levels • Good for indigestion • Reduces menstrual pain • Lowers cholesterol levels • Possesses anti-cancerous properties • Protects against alzhemiers • Fights infections • Boosts the immune system
Peppermint	• Soothes the stomach • Nausea • Anti-microbial • Anti-cancerous properties • Aids ease of breathing • Irritable Bowel Syndrome (IBS)

Cloves	• Soothes toothache • Nausea • Relieves respiratory infection symptoms • Anti-inflammatory • Digestion • Sooths cuts and bruises
Cumin	• Nausea • Lowers blood sugar levels • Lowers cholesterol levels • Boosts the immune system • Good for bone health • Digestion • Anti-cancerous properties
Fennel	• Nausea • Digestion • Anaemia • Flatulence • Heart health • Lowers blood pressure levels • Anti-cancerous properties • Menstrual issues • Brain health • Diarrhoea • Colic
Baking Soda	• Skin health • Heartburn and indigestion • Ulcer relief • Good for sunburn • Teeth whitener
Tea Tree Oil	• Skin health • Softens cuticles • Good for sores • Dry skin

	<ul><li>Skin tag removal</li><li>Hair growth</li><li>Anti-dandruff</li><li>Dry scalp</li><li>Prevents hair fall</li><li>Fights bacterial and viral infections</li></ul>
Avocado Soybean Unsaponifiables (ASU)	<ul><li>Arthritis</li><li>Lowers cholesterol</li></ul>
Black Currant Oil (Ribes Nigrum)	<ul><li>Arthritis</li><li>Digestion</li><li>Helps night vision</li><li>Digestion</li></ul>
Evening Primrose	<ul><li>Arthritis</li><li>Helps to improve diabetic related nerve damage</li><li>Strengthens bones</li></ul>
Fish Oil	<ul><li>Arthritis</li><li>Lower triglycerides</li><li>Heart health</li><li>Anxiety</li><li>Reduces Alzheimer's symptoms</li><li>Anti-cancerous properties</li><li>Improves ADHD (Attention Deficit Hyperactivity Disorder)</li></ul>
Garlic	<ul><li>Lowers blood pressure</li><li>Fights cold and flu symptoms</li><li>Reduces cholesterol levels</li><li>Improves Alzheimer symptoms</li><li>Detoxifies the body</li><li>Improves bone health</li></ul>
Ginger	<ul><li>Reduce high blood pressure</li><li>Reduces nausea</li><li>Reduces muscle pain and soreness</li></ul>

	• General tonic • Anti-inflammatory • Lowers blood sugar levels • Improves digestion • Reduces menstrual pain • Possesses anti-cancerous properties • Fights infections • Improves brain health
Cardamom	• Improves blood pressure levels • Aids digestion • Relieves stomach acidity levels • Helps relieve respiratory infection symptoms • Regulates heart rate • Fights anaemia • Detoxifies the body • Improves sexual performance
Rauvolfia Serpentine	• High blood pressure • Anxiety • Schizophrenia • Verigo • Giddiness • Snakebite
Bilberry Extract	• Strengthens blood vessels • Improves circulation • Helps fight retinopathy
Fenugreek	• Diabetes • Lowers cholesterol • Relieves heart burn • Reduces menstrual symptoms • Reduces cholesterol levels
Black Cohosh	• Menopausal symptoms • Muscle cramps

	• Insomnia • Headaches
Soy	• Menopausal symptoms • Reduces breast and endometrial cancer • Helps bone health • Heart health • Boosts cognitive function
Ginseng	• Menopausal symptoms • Reduces blood sugar levels • Boosts memory owner • Improves ADHD (Attention Deficit Hyperactivity Disorder) • Fights cold and flu symptoms • Anti-cancerous properties • Boosts sexual performance • General tonic

Footnotes

Chapter Two – Anxiety

1.   Jerome Sarris, Con Stough, Chad A. Bousman, Zahra T. Wahid, Greg Murray, Rolf Teschke, Karen M. Savage, Ashley Dowell, Chee Ng, Isaac Schweitzer. Kava in the Treatment of Generalized Anxiety Disorder.Journal of Clinical Psychopharmacology, 2013; 1 DOI:

2.   Hyperforin, the active component of St. John's wort, induces IL-8 expression in human intestinal epithelial cells via a MAPK-dependent, NF-kappaB-independent pathway.

Zhou C1, Tabb MM, Sadatrafiei A, Grün F, Sun A, Blumberg B.

3.   Laakmann G, Schule C, Baghai T, et al. St. John's wort in mild to moderate depression: the relevance of hyperforin for the clinical efficacy. Pharmacopsychiat 1998; 31(suppl): 54-59.]

4.   Zaichikova SG, Grinkevich NI, Barabanov EI, et al. Healing properties and determination of the upper parameters of toxicity of Hypericum herb. Farmatsiya. 1985;34:62-64.

5.   Barbagallo C, Chisari G. Antimicrobial activity of three hypericum species.Fitoterapia. 1987;58:175-180.

6.   Razinkov SP, Yerofeyeva LN, Khovrina MP, Lazarev AI. Validation of the use of Hypericum perforatum medicamentous form with a prolonged action to treat patients with maxillary sinusitis. Zh Ushn Nos Gorl Bolezn. 1989;49:43-46.

7.   Martinez B, Kasper S, Ruhrmann S, Moller H-J. Hypericum in the treatment of seasonal affective disorders. Nervenheilkunde. 1993;12:302-307.

8.   Valerenic acid potentiates and inhibits GABAA receptors: Molecular mechanism and subunit specificity

S. Khoma, I. Baburina, E. Timina, A. Hohausa, G. Traunerb, B. Koppb, S. Heringa, ,

9.   Valerian extract and valerenic acid are partial agonists of the 5-HT5a receptor in vitro

Birgit M. Dietza, b, Gail B. Mahadya, b, , , Guido F. Paulib, Norman R. Farnsworthb

10.   Pharmacopsychiatry. 2000 Mar;33(2):47-53.

Critical evaluation of the effect of valerian extract on sleep structure and sleep quality.

Donath F1, Quispe S, Diefenbach K, Maurer A, Fietze I, Roots I.

148

11.   Passionflower in the treatment of generalized anxiety: a pilot double-blind randomized controlled trial with oxazepam

S. Akhondzadeh PhD1,2, H. R. Naghavi MD1, M. Vazirian MD1, A. Shayeganpour PharmD2,

H. Rashidi PharmD2 andM. Khani MSc2

 Article first published online: 12 JAN 2002

DOI: 10.1046/j.1365-2710.2001.00367.x

12.   Planta Med. 1995 Jun;61(3):213-6.

Apigenin, a component of Matricaria recutita flowers, is a central benzodiazepine receptors-ligand with anxiolytic effects.

Viola H1, Wasowski C, Levi de Stein M, Wolfman C, Silveira R, Dajas F, Medina JH, Paladini AC.

Chapter Three – Allergies

1.   Randomised controlled trial of butterbur and cetirizine for treating seasonal allergic rhinitis

BMJ 2002; 324 doi: http://dx.doi.org/10.1136/bmj.324.7330.144 (Published 19 January 2002)Cite this as: BMJ 2002;324:144

2.   Biochem Pharmacol. 2001 Apr 15;61(8):1041-7.

Role of petasin in the potential anti-inflammatory activity of a plant extract of petasites hybridus.

Thomet OA1, Wiesmann UN, Schapowal A, Bizer C, Simon HU.

3.   Lipton RB, Göbel, H,Einhäupl KM, et al. Petasites hybridus root (butterbur) is an effective preventive treatment for migraine. Neurology, 2004;63:2240-4.

4.   Butterbur, a herbal remedy, confers complementary anti-inflammatory activity in asthmatic patients receiving inhaled corticosteroids

Authors: D. K. C. Lee,K. Haggart,F. M. Robb,B. J. Lipworth : First published: 14 January 2004.

5.   J Allergy Clin Immunol. 1984 Jun;73(6):801-9.

149

Flavonoid modulation of human neutrophil function.

Busse WW, Kopp DE, Middleton E Jr.

6.   Nettle extract (Urtica dioica) affects key receptors and enzymes associated with allergic rhinitis

Bill Roschek Jr.1, Ryan C. Fink2, Matthew McMichael1 andRandall S. Alberte1,*

Article first published online: 12 JAN 2009   DOI: 10.1002/ptr.2763

7.   Randomized, double-blind study of freeze-dried Urtica dioica in the treatment of allergic rhinitis.

(PMID:2192379)

Mittman P

National College of Naturopathic Medicine, Portland, Oregon 97216.

Planta Medica [1990, 56(1):44-47]

Type: Clinical Trial, Journal Article, Randomized Controlled Trial

Chapter Four – Cold and Flu

1.   Efficacy and tolerability of a fluid extract combination of thyme herb and ivy leaves and matched placebo in adults suffering from acute bronchitis with productive cough. A prospective, double-blind, placebo-controlled clinical trial.

(PMID:17063641)

Kemmerich B , Eberhardt R , Stammer H

Practice for Internal Medicine and Pneumology, Munich, Germany.

Arzneimittel-Forschung [2006, 56(9):652-660]

Type: Journal Article, Randomized Controlled Trial

2.   Kong F. Pilot clinical study on a proprietary elderberry extract: efficacy in addressing influenza symptoms. Online Journal of Pharmacology and Pharmacokinetics.2009;5:32-43.

3.   Jostling PD. Preventing the common cold with garlic supplement contains allicin: A double blind, placebo controlled survey. Advance in Therapy; Volume 18 No.4

4.   Effect of Natural Honey (Produced by African sculata in Guyana) Against Bacteria (Pseudomonas aeruginosa, Escherichia coli and Staphylococcus aureus) and Fungus (Candida albicans)

AA Ansari, C Alexander - World Journal of Dairy & Food Sciences, 2009 - idosi.org

5.   Natural Honey Lowers Plasma Glucose, C-Reactive Protein, Homocysteine, and Blood Lipids in Healthy, Diabetic, and Hyperlipidemic Subjects: Comparison with Dextrose and Sucrose

Noori S. Al-Waili. Journal of Medicinal Food. July 2004, 7(1): 100-107. doi:10.1089/109662004322984789

6.   J Nat Prod. 1994 May;57(5):658-62.

Isolation of antirhinoviral sesquiterpenes from ginger (Zingiber officinale).

Denyer CV1, Jackson P, Loakes DM, Ellis MR, Young DA.

Chapter Five – Headaches

1.   EFFECTS OF SEVERAL MONOAMINE OXIDASE INHIBITORS ON THE CARDIOVASCULAR ACTIONS OF NATURALLY OCCURRING AMINES IN THE DOG

Leon I. Goldberg and Albert Sjoerdsma

J Pharmacol Exp Ther November 1959 127:178-181; published onlineNovember 1, 1959

2.   Migraine Prevention in Children and Adolescents: Results of an Open Study With a Special Butterbur Root Extract

R Pothmann, U Danesch - Headache: The Journal of Head and …, 2005 - Wiley Online Library

151

3.   Petasites hybridus root (butterbur) is an effective preventive treatment for migraine

R. B. Lipton, MD, H. Göbel, MD, PhD, K. M. Einhäupl, MD, K. Wilks, MD and A. Mauskop, MD

4.   Efficacy and safety of 6.25 mg t.i.d. feverfew CO2-extract (MIG-99) in migraine prevention – a randomized, double-blind, multicentre, placebo-controlled study

HC Diener1,*, V Pfaffenrath2, J Schnitker3,M Friede4, H-H Henneicke-von Zepelin4andthe Investigators1

Article first published online: 13 MAY 2005   DOI: 10.1111/j.1468-2982.2005.00950.x

5.   Response of Cluster Headache to Kudzu

R. Andrew Sewell MD

Article first published online: 9 OCT 2008

DOI: 10.1111/j.1526-4610.2008.01268.x

© 2008 the Author. Journal compilation © 2008 American Headache Society

6.   Therapy for Acute Nonpurulent Rhinosinusitis With Cineole: Results of a Double-Blind, Randomized, Placebo-Controlled Trial†

Wolfgang Kehrl MD1,*, Uwe Sonnemann MD2 andUwe Dethlefsen PhD3

Article first published online: 3 JAN 2009

DOI: 10.1097/00005537-200404000-00027

Chapter Six – Stomach

1.   Infect Control Hosp Epidemiol. 2000 Jan;21(1):33-8.

Antimicrobial activity of home disinfectants and natural products against potential human pathogens.

152

Rutala WA1, Barbee SL, Aguiar NC, Sobsey MD, Weber DJ.

2.   Aloe vera gel in peptic ulcer therapy; Preliminary report

JJ Blitz, JW Smith, JR Gerard - Journal AOA, 1963 - blog.samlennon.net

Chapter Seven – Nausea

1.   Ginger for Nausea and Vomiting in Pregnancy: Randomized, Double-Masked, Placebo-Controlled Trial

VUTYAVANICH, TERAPORN MD, MSC; KRAISARIN, THEERAJANA MD; RUANGSRI, RUNG-AROON BSC.

2.   Peppermint oil: a treatment for postoperative nausea

Sylvina Tate MSc BSc (Hons) RGN DipN PGDE RNT*

Article first published online: 28 JUN 2008

DOI: 10.1046/j.1365-2648.1997.t01-15-00999.x

3.   The Effect of Lemon Inhalation Aromatherapy on Nausea and Vomiting of Pregnancy: A Double-Blinded, Randomized, Controlled Clinical Trial

Parisa Yavari kia,1 Farzaneh Safajou,1,* Mahnaz Shahnazi,1 and Hossein Nazemiyeh2

Author information ▶ Article notes ▶ Copyright and License information ▶

Chapter Eight – Acne and Skin

1.   A comparative study of tea-tree oil versus benzoylperoxide in the treatment of acne

Bassett IB , Pannowitz DL , Barnetson RS

Department of Dermatology, Royal Prince Alfred Hospital, Camperdown, NSW.

The Medical Journal of Australia [1990, 153(8):455-458]

Type: Clinical Trial, Journal Article, Randomized Controlled Trial, Comparative Study

Chapter Nine - Arthritis

1.   Avocado/soybean unsaponifiables increase aggrecan synthesis and reduce catabolic and proinflammatory mediator production by human osteoarthritic chondrocytes.

Yves E Henrotin, Christelle Sanchez, Michelle A Deberg, Nathalie Piccardi,

Georges Bernard Guillou, Philippe Msika, and Jean-Yves L Reginster

Journal of Rheumatology, 2003 - jrheum.org

2.   Symptomatic efficacy of avocado–soybean unsaponifiables (ASU) in osteoarthritis (OA) patients: a meta-analysis of randomized controlled trials 1

R. Christensen, M.Sc.†, E.M. Bartels, D.Sc.†, ‡, A. Astrup, M.D., Ph.D.§, H. Bliddal, M.D., Ph.D.†

3.   Gamma-linolenic acid treatment of rheumatoid arthritis. A randomized, placebo-controlled trial

Robert B. Zurier MD1,*, Ronald G. Rossetti MPH1, Eric W. Jacobson MD1, Deborah M. Demarco MD1, Nancy Y. Liu MD1, Joseph E. Temming MD1, Bernadette M. White RN1andMichael Laposata MD, PhD2

Article first published online: 12 DEC 2005

DOI: 10.1002/art.1780391106

4.   Fish-Oil Fatty Acid Supplementation in Active Rheumatoid Arthritis: A Double-Blinded, Controlled, Crossover Study

JOEL M. KREMER, M.D.; WILLIAM JUBIZ, M.D.; ANN MICHALEK, M.D.; RICHARD I. RYNES, M.D.; LEE E. BARTHOLOMEW, M.D.; JEAN BIGAOUETTE, R.D.; MARYANN TIMCHALK, B.S.; DONALD BEELER, Ph.D.; and LLOYD LININGER, Ph.D.

[+] Article, Author, and Disclosure Information

154

Ann Intern Med. 1987;106(4):497-503. doi:10.7326/0003-4819-106-4-497

Chapter Ten – High Blood Pressure

1. Glycated haemoglobin and blood pressure-lowering effect of cinnamon in multi-ethnic Type 2 diabetic patients in the UK: a randomized, placebo-controlled, double-blind clinical trial

R. Akilen, A. Tsiami, D. Devendra andN. Robinson

Article first published online: 5 JUL 2010

DOI: 10.1111/j.1464-5491.2010.03079.x

© 2010 The Authors. Diabetic Medicine © 2010 Diabetes UK

2.   Effects of Cinnamon Consumption on Glycemic Status, Lipid Profile and Body Composition in Type 2 Diabetes Patients

Vafa, Mohammad Reza; Mohammadi, Farhad; Shidfar, Farzad; Mohammadhossein Salehi Sormaghi; Heidari, Iraj; et al. International Journal of Preventive Medicine 3.8 (Aug 2012): n/a.

3.   Effect of garlic on blood pressure: A systematic review and meta-analysis

Karin RiedEmail author, Oliver R Frank, Nigel P Stocks, Peter Fakler and Thomas Sullivan

BMC Cardiovascular Disorders20088:13

DOI: 10.1186/1471-2261-8-13

© Ried et al. 2008

Received: 26 March 2008

Accepted: 16 June 2008

Published: 16 June 2008

4.   Effect of allicin from garlic powder on serum lipids and blood pressure in rats fed with a high cholesterol diet

M. Ali, K.K. Al-Qattan, F. Al-Enezi, R.M.A. Khanafer, T. Mustafa

155

DOI: http://dx.doi.org/10.1054/plef.2000.0152

5.   J Cardiovasc Pharmacol. 2005 Jan;45(1):74-80.

Ginger lowers blood pressure through blockade of voltage-dependent calcium channels.

Ghayur MN1, Gilani AH.

6.   [PDF] Blood pressure lowering, fibrinolysis enhancing and antioxidant activities of cardamom(Elettaria cardamomum)

SK Verma, V Jain, SS Katewa - Indian journal of biochemistry & ..., 2009 - researchgate.net

7.   A CLINICAL TRIAL OF RAUWOLFIA SERPENTINA IN ESSENTIAL HYPERTENSION / RUSTOM JAL VAKIL/ Cardiological Department, King Edward Memorial Hospital, Bombay, India / Jan 1949

8.   Mechanism of Hypotensive Action of Reserpine, an Alkaloid of Rauwolfia serpentina

E. G. MCQUEEN, A. E. DOYLE & F. H. SMIRK

Department of Medicine, Otago University Medical School, Dunedin, New Zealand. July 20.

Chapter Eleven - Diabetes

1.   [PDF] CINNAMON, CARDAMOM AND GINGER IMPACTS AS EVALUATED ON HYPERGLYCEMIC RATS.

MA El-yamani - J. of specific education, 2011 - mans.edu.eg

2.   Effects of a cinnamon extract on plasma glucose, HbA1c, and serum lipids in diabetes mellitus type 2

B. Mang1, M. Wolters1, B. Schmitt1, K. Kelb1, R. Lichtinghagen2, D. O. Stichtenoth2 andA. Hahn1Article first published online: 18 APR 2006

DOI: 10.1111/j.1365-2362.2006.01629.x

156

3.   Beneficial effects of Aloe vera leaf gel extract on lipid profile status in rats with streptozotocindiabetes

S Rajasekaran, K Ravi, K Sivagnanam… - Clinical and …, 2006 - Wiley Online Library

4.   Antidiabetic activity of Aloe vera L. juice II. Clinical trial in diabetes mellitus patients in combination with glibenclamide

N. Bunyapraphatsara1, *, S. Yongchaiyudha1, V. Rungpitarangsi2, O. Chokechaijaroenporn2

1 Medicinal Plant Information Center, Faculty of Pharmacy, Mahidol University

2 Department of Preventive and Social Medicine, Faculty of Medicine Siriraj Hospital, Mahidol University

5.   Influence of aloe vera on the healing of dermal wounds in diabetic rats

P Chithra, G.B Sajithlal, Gowri Chandrakasan

Department of Biochemistry, Central Leather Research Institute, Adyar, Chennai 600 020, IndiaReceived 18 August 1997, Revised 6 October 1997, Accepted 12 October 1997, Available online 4 March 1999

6.   Endocrine, Visual and Auditory Systems Vision preservation during retinal inflammation by anthocyanin-rich bilberry extract: cellular and molecular mechanism

Seiji Miyake1,2,3, Noriko Takahashi1,2, Mariko Sasaki1,2, Saori Kobayashi3, Kazuo Tsubota1 and Yoko Ozawa1,2

1Laboratory of Retinal Cell Biology, Keio University School of Medicine, Tokyo, Japan

2Department of Ophthalmology, Keio University School of Medicine, Tokyo, Japan

3Wakasa Seikatsu, Kyoto, Japan

7.   J Appl Physiol (1985). 2006 Apr;100(4):1164-70. Epub 2005 Dec 8.

Direct vasoactive and vasoprotective properties of anthocyanin-rich extracts.

Bell DR1, Gochenaur K.

8.   Perossini M, Guidi G, Chiellini S, Siravo D. Diabetic and hypertensive retinopathy therapy with Vaccinium myrtillus anthocyanosides (Tegens®): Double-blind, placebo-controlled clinical trial. Ann Ottalmol Clin Ocul1987;113:1173-7 [in Italian].

157

9.   Effect of Trigonella foenum-graecum (fenugreek) seeds on glycaemic control and insulin resistance in type 2 diabetes mellitus: a double blind placebo controlled study.

(PMID:11868855)

Gupta A , Gupta R , Lal B

Jaipur Diabetes and Research Centre.

The Journal of the Association of Physicians of India [2001, 49:1057-1061]

Type: Clinical Trial, Journal Article, Randomized Controlled Trial, Comparative Study

10.   Keen H, Payan J, Allawi J, et al. Treatment of diabetic neuropathy with gamma-linolenic acid. The gamma-Linolenic Acid Multicenter Trial Group. Diabetes Care. 1993;16:8-15. abstract: www.ncbi.nlm.nih.gov/pubmed/8380765

Chapter Twelve - Menopause

1.   The Cimicifuga preparation BNO 1055 vs. conjugated estrogens in a double-blind placebo-controlled study: effects on menopause symptoms and bone markers

W Wuttkea, , , D Seidlová-Wuttkea, C Gorkowb

Maturitas

Volume 44, Supplement, 14 March 2003, Pages S67–S77

Modern Phytotherapy in Menopause: Cimicifuga racemosa (Klimadynon, Menofem) Pharmacological and Clinical Data, June 10th 2002, Berlin

2.   Geller SE, Shulman LP, van Breemen RB, Banuvar S, Zhou

Y, Epstein G, et al.Safety and efficacy of black cohosh and red clover for the management of vasomotor symptoms:

a randomised controlled trial. Menopause 2009;16(6):

1156–66.

158

3.		Obstetrics & Gynecology:

March 2002 – Volume 99-Issue 3- p389-394

Original Research

Benefits of Soy Isoflavone Therapeutic Regimen on Menopausal Symptoms

Han, Kyung K. MD; Soares, Jose M. Jr MD; Haidar, Mauro A. MD, PhD; de Lima, Geraldo Rodrigues MD, PhD; Baracat, Edmund C. MD, PhD

4.		January 2001 - Volume 8 - Issue 1 - pp 17-26

Isoflavone-rich or isoflavone-poor soy protein does not reduce menopausal symptoms during 24 weeks of treatment

St. Germain, Alison MS, RD1; Peterson, Charles T. MS2; Robinson, Jennifer G. MD, MPH3; Alekel, D. Lee PhD, RD1

5.		Menopause:

April 2012 - Volume 19 - Issue 4 - p 461–466

doi: 10.1097/gme.0b013e3182325e4b

Original Articles

Effects of red ginseng supplementation on menopausal symptoms and cardiovascular risk factors in postmenopausal women: a double-blind randomized controlled trial

Kim, Sun Young MD1; Seo, Seok Kyo MD2; Choi, Young Mi MD2; Jeon, Young Eun MD1; Lim, Kyung Jin MD2; Cho, SiHyun MD1; Choi, Young Sik MD2; Lee, Byung Seok MD, PhD1

Notes

www.ingramcontent.com/pod-product-compliance
Lightning Source LLC
Chambersburg PA
CBHW060312290526
45789CB00001B/492

* 9 7 8 1 5 3 7 6 0 1 2 4 3 *